MW00979851

If There's Nothing Wrong With Me, Then Why Do I Feel So Bad?

Dr. Ric Arseneau
604-417-5194
CPSBC 13459, MSP 09308

If There's Nothing Wrong With Me, Then Why Do I Feel So Bad?

▼

The Neurologic Basis of Fibromyalgia, Chronic Fatigue Syndrome and Related Disorders

Martin A. Duclos, MD

Writer's Showcase

New York Lincoln Shanghai

If There's Nothing Wrong With Me, Then Why Do I Feel So Bad?
The Neurologic Basis of Fibromyalgia,
Chronic Fatigue Syndrome and Related Disorders

All Rights Reserved © 2002 by Martin A. Duclos

No part of this book may be reproduced or transmitted in any form or by any means, graphic, electronic, or mechanical, including photocopying, recording, taping, or by any information storage retrieval system, without the written permission of the publisher.

Writer's Showcase
an imprint of iUniverse, Inc.

For information address:
iUniverse
2021 Pine Lake Road, Suite 100
Lincoln, NE 68512
www.iuniverse.com

The enclosed information is educational in nature and not as substitute for appropriate medical care.

ISBN: 0-595-24849-7

Printed in the United States of America

Dedication

Without the ability of my wife Anna to run a household, raise three children, and maintain a rapidly growing psychiatric office practice while I sat in my basement at the word processor, this book would not have been possible. She has been my inspiration, my friend, and the enduring love of my life. I also want to thank my children, Jeffrey Christian, Matthew Andrew, and Abigail Rose, who are too young to understand what daddy was doing down there in the basement, but who didn't bother me down there, much. I owe a debt of gratitude for the support of my colleagues at Edward Jew III and Associates and to Peter Adams and others at Highmark Blue Cross and Blue Shield who encouraged me when they could have discouraged me, proving that they value patient care and medical education above all else. Lastly, I want to thank my patients, who have taught me much more about these disorders than all the medical textbooks in the world could have.

Contents

Foreword

There are many things that this book tries to accomplish, and there are many things it is not. I have tried to provide an overview of a very complicated subject called Somatoneural Dysfunction. It is a subject that very few physicians and professors understand and one that, despite studying clinically for the last ten years, I learn something new about every day. I have provided a historical overview in chapter 1, mainly in order to illustrate the medical community's theories and errors in attempting to understand the problem of SND.

SND is not chronic fatigue syndrome, nor is it fibromyalgia, nor any other of a host of interrelated disorders. Rather it is all of them and none of them at the same time. These syndromes do, however, share certain characteristics that will hopefully become apparent. Therefore I prefer to focus on these similarities in order to explain a syndrome that makes patients miserable, but fails to fit into a well-defined set of illnesses in the medical realm.

In order to understand a problem this complicated, we need to learn some mechanisms of health and disease. Before understanding of a pathologic state can occur, we need to know how the darn thing should operate under healthy circumstances. All too often, physicians forget this and fail to explain either how the system functions normally or why it has malfunctioned adequately to patients.

Hopefully, the information provided in chapter 2 and expanded upon later on in the text will be relatively easy to comprehend. I have written this book in a style at the level of a medical student and provided frequent addendums to clarify points that may be particularly complex. I have chosen not to "dumb down" this information simply because you, the reader, have not gone to medical school. Rather I have attempted to bring your level of understanding up a bit, and if, after reading it, you do wish to go to medical school (after realizing it's not that tough after all), please let me know!

This book describes SND and its related syndromes in regards to ongoing clinical and basic science research. It attempts to provide a framework of understanding of the disease process so that when we get to treatments in Part 2, you will know why these things may work and why they may not. Discussion of the psychological aspects of health and illness in general and with regards to SND in particular can be found here as well. This is an area that is critical to understand in fully grasping this disorder and assisting with therapy. Unfortunately, through association with bad connotations and misunderstanding, it is the area most neglected and overlooked.

Somatoneural Dysfunction is a name that indicates the abnormality in the way sensory information is processed in patients with fibromyalgia and other related syndromes. Thus, it should be qualified as a neurologic disorder. This makes a lot of sense because of the way the central nervous system interacts with and affects every other organ system in the body.

That is what this is, and I thank you for reading at least this far. Let me take a brief moment to also tell you what this book is not.

1) A pop psychology text: I am not here to tell you that thinking happy thoughts will cure you. That is not to say that thinking happy thoughts does not have a role in the treatment of Somatoneural Dysfunction and other disorders, however, and I encourage everyone to think only happy thoughts always.

2)   A research text: although it certainly contains enough references to research, I am a practicing physician and have long since forgotten which end of a Bunsen burner to light. We owe a great debt to basic and clinical science researchers, but need to evaluate their theories and findings in terms of patient care. That is what I do. Every day. And on weekends. And sometimes in the middle of the night.

3)   An alternative medicine text: I believe in a union of alternative and traditional medicine in treating many disorders, and the understanding of Somatoneural Dysfunction is no exception. I believe the mainstream medical community is wrong to have ignored this area of potential benefit for the last century. I also believe that use of alternative therapies without proof by research is dangerous. Everything "natural" is not necessarily good, safe, and effective. Cyanide is natural. Black widow spiders are natural.

So with all that in mind, I hope you will continue to read, to learn, to question, and to believe that there is hope for the millions and millions of patients who still feel miserable, even though their doctors tell them not to. Whether you have been diagnosed with chronic fatigue syndrome or fibromyalgia, or ever been told by a doctor that your symptoms are "all in your head", this book will attempt to answer your questions and explain why the medical community has been so wrong for so many years in this important area.

When you are convinced that you have Somatoneural Dysfunction (in whichever its manifestations) and you understand what is going on in your body by the end of this book, you will be ready to start a specific treatment program designed to limit symptoms and recondition your body and mind. That comes in part 2.

Introduction

Mrs. J. M. was a sixty-four year old housewife who came to my community office practice one afternoon in 1998. She was a striking lady with chiseled features and bright blue eyes that sparkled with a hidden life. The rest of her face, however, was deeply lined with wrinkles making her look ten or twenty years older than she actually was. She had come to see me upon the request of her niece, who was another patient of mine, hoping against all hope that I would be able to diagnose her illness and provide some long overdue relief from her symptoms.

She had forwarded her medical records to me earlier and I had perused them at some length a few days prior to our scheduled appointment. They were quite voluminous, spanning visits to a myriad of doctors, specialists, and hospitals, and covered endless physicals, blood tests, imaging studies, and treatment failures. Her problems seemed to start in the late seventies, a year or so after the death of her husband to skin cancer. Her doctors initially attributed her profound fatigue, headaches, and stomach pains to stress and grieving.

Eventually, she was referred to a nationally renowned hospital, where they performed CAT scans of her brain and abdomen, about a thousand blood tests, many of which had been done on more than one occasion previously, and even a procedure where they put a needle into her spinal canal to remove cerebrospinal fluid for analysis. She was told all her tests were negative and reached the same conclusion as her previous doctors, that she suffered from stress and depression.

Therefore, she was started on Valium™ for her stress and phenobarbital to prevent her headaches. No one would treat her for depression until she was finally referred to a psychiatrist in 1995, nearly fifteen years after her symptoms had started. She became, predictably, addicted to the phenobarbital and struggled with that for nearly eight years. The Valium™ she remained on for nearly a decade until our visit, without any evidence that it was at all beneficial.

A neurologist told her she had migraines, a gastroenterologist diagnosed spastic colon after looking down into her stomach and up into her colon with endoscopes, and a rheumatologist thought the aches and pains in her joints were from rheumatoid arthritis. Despite persistently negative blood tests and x-rays, he placed her on gold injections and hydroxychloroquine, which provided no relief, but did make her hair fall out. She had palpitations and a cardiologist thought he heard a prolapsed mitral valve. I didn't hear one, and neither did the echocardiogram I obtained, thus allowing her to end her yearly ritual of taking a handful of antibiotics every six months before her teeth cleanings.

Around 1994, she began to pursue alternative medicine practitioners due to the inability of the medical profession to provide any answers. She dabbled in aromatherapy, tried acupuncture, and visited a chiropractor, who claimed all her complaints were from a malalignment in the vertebral bodies of her back. She had never had trouble with her back, she protested, but did develop low back pain after a series of spinal manipulations he performed. A Chinese herbalist gave her ginseng and dong quai, which made her constipated, and another practitioner cleansed her colon with enemas, claiming to remove all the evil humors. He did not succeed, apparently, but did fix the constipation caused by the ginseng and dong quai.

So it was little wonder that she did not hold much faith that I, a little less than a year in practice, wound be able to help her. As we spoke, however, she came to realize that not only did I believe that I knew what she had, and not only had I seen dozens of other patients with problems just like hers, but that I thought I could provide some insight into her treatment. Her bright blue eyes sparkled at that, but darkened again when I said that I could not cure her or even guarantee that I could make her feel better. A seed of hope was planted there, however, as I explained that the power to treat this ailment would come mainly from within herself.

In the rest of this book I will attempt to explain this illness, that some have labeled chronic fatigue syndrome, fibromyalgia, idiopathic chronic fatigue, myofascial pain syndrome, and many other things. All of these definitions fall a bit short though, as I will explain. I have called this condition Somatoneural Dysfunction (SND) for the sake of convenience and nomenclature, but I must caution that the constellation of symptoms and effective treatments are highly variable.

Chapter 1:
Modern and Historical Perspectives

The Definition

Let's start with a working definition of Somatoneural Dysfunction. "Somato" refers to the body and "Neural" to the brain and central nervous system. Thus Somatoneural Dysfunction refers to a malfunction in the way sensory information from the body is interpreted by the brain. Usually this results in a hypersensitivity of the CNS, but may produce abnormal interpretation of the sensory input as well. For example, a sprained ankle may result in excruciating pain that last for weeks if a patient has SND, or may lead to an abnormal burning or numbing sensation all the way up the leg.

In my own clinical practice I resist giving this disorder a more specific name or a set of characteristic signs and symptoms simply because the presentation is so different from patient to patient. Most patients with the diffuse symptoms of overwhelming fatigue and chronic aches and pains do not fit nicely into a single category such as fibromyalgia or chronic fatigue syndrome.

Why do physicians and medical researchers continually try to cram patients into these well-defined categories? Well, it may be force of habit from the way doctors learn medicine. In medical school, students are expected to learn an enormous amount of information and it is simply easier to split the information into discrete packages of data to memorize. This is called chunking. It's also partly due to the constraints of clinical research, which has historically focused on patients with very similar syndromes in order to standardize the results.

With regards to Somatoneural Dysfunction, the medical profession has attempted for decades to categorize patients into narrow subdivisions in order to research the cause and come up with effective treatments. Unfortunately, we had one group that was working on Gulf War Syndrome in California, another studying chronic fatigue syndrome in Minnesota, and a third looking at fibromyalgia in New York. All this and more was done without ever realizing that it is the similarities between the syndromes and not the differences that hold the key to better understanding.

This has all led to a great deal of confusion among patients and doctors alike. The medical profession has, for some reason, held onto the belief that a single biological defect can cause such a variety of symptom complexes. I believe that an abnormally sensitive central nervous system is at the root of Somatoneural Dysfunction and is responsible for each of the similar clinical syndromes we will discuss. There are two main reasons why the reluctance to accept this rationale is unfounded:

1) We now know that the central nervous system interacts directly and indirectly with every other organ system in the body and can be responsible for virtually every symptom presentation possible.
2) Many other diseases and disorders have extremely varied clinical presentations as well. Lupus, for example, can range from a mild skin disease to a crippling, lethal syndrome of multiple organ failure

I continue to stress to my patients that SND affects each person differently. When a patient named Jones asks me what exactly the heck it is that makes him feel so darn tired all the time, I tell him it is Jones' Disease. Another important point to remember is that Jones' Disease is treated differently than Jackson's Disease or Ramirez's Disease. This may seem like a surprising concept to many patients and doctors, but it is how good medicine has been practiced for centuries. Ayurvedic physicians who have developed their system of medicine in India over the last three-thousand years say that they never try to figure out what kind of illness a person has, rather, they spend their time trying to determine what kind of person has the illness. This is similar to Chinese medical philosophy and holistic medicine. Chinese practitioners believe that disease stems from an imbalance in the body's energy and life forces while holistic theory focuses on stress to the body as a disruption of the natural state of harmony that maintains health.

That is not to say that studying small groups of patients with similar clinical features is not useful. In fact, it is extremely useful and the basis for all medical treatment. The art of medicine comes in determining whether the results of a particular study apply to a given patient. That is a far cry from the "cookbook" approach to medicine that has flourished in recent years.

Therefore I have tried to illustrate the abnormalities in Somatoneural Dysfunction in broad strokes that take into account the individual differences in the disorder. I will provide you with some common features of SND, each of which will be explained in more detail. This can help determine if this problem applies to you or someone you know.

The common thread of Somatoneural Dysfunction is fatigue. Usually the fatigue is like the dullness of a toothache, making it difficult to work, exercise, and enjoy life to the fullest. Sometimes this fatigue becomes pervasive and overwhelming, but more often it just lies there dormant, like a snarling old dog. Often, the fatigue worsens with exertion, and may become exhausting with the simplest activities like climbing a flight of stair or doing the laundry. The lack of energy that accompanies the fatigue can make it difficult to get through the day. In certain patients, this is the only symptom of SND, and this is sometimes referred to as Chronic Idiopathic Fatigue. This is doctor-speak for "fatigue that has been there a long time and we don't know what caused it".

The problems that can accompany this fatigue, as I have mentioned, may involve any organ system in the body. Common manifestations include: headache, memory and concentration impairment, muscle and joint aches and pains, irritable bowels with diarrhea or constipation, dizziness or lightheadedness, palpitations, poor sleep or insomnia which results in feeling unrefreshed upon waking, tingling or numbness in the hands or feet, the sensation of swollen or tight hands, stomach upset, chronic cough, and premenstrual cramping.

Wow. That sure covers a lot of ground, and it has only scratched the surface of the problem. Individual patients can have any, all, or none of those symptoms, but in all cases, the fatigue is the underlying clue to the problem. If this sounds like you, read on. In fact, even if it doesn't, read on anyway, because this approach to dealing with health and illness is somewhat unique and may be applicable to many other medical problems as well. I have combined a holistic approach to identification of the problem with traditional medical theory and treatment planning, sprinkling in alternative practices where they are safe and potentially effective. This method of medical practice is called "integrative medicine" and is without a doubt the medicine of the new millennium not only to apply to Somatoneural Dysfunction, but to all medical fields.

Finally, we must come to the understanding that psychiatric factors play a major role in the pathogenesis and treatment of Somatoneural Dysfunction. Wait, before you put this book back down and head over to the Stephen King section, listen to a stunning revelation. Psychiatric factors play a major role in EVERY medical problem. The problem is that patients don't like to admit this and doctors don't know how to address the issue themselves.

I hope to convince you that this is true, that psychiatric factors do play a role in SND, but more importantly I want to provide the insight that this is not a bad thing. It is also something that we can use to our distinct advantage in outlining a comprehensive plan of attack in treating sufferers with SND. A positive attitude has been proven to help in the treatment of many medical disorders, and Somatoneural Dysfunction is no exception.

The Scope of the Problem

What we do know about Somatoneural Dysfunction is that it has perplexed medical investigators for centuries and has presented itself in a variety of ways. I would estimate that SND affects up to 25% of the US population at some time or another during the course of their lives. If we look at fatigue alone, the one symptom that is usually present in all types of SND, 24% of the general adult population has experienced profound fatigue lasting longer than two weeks and necessitating consultation with a health care provider (Price, 1992). One estimate noted that 24% of primary care clinic patients reported having had fatigue lasting longer than four weeks at some point in the preceding year (Kroenke, 1988). Nearly half of these patients with prolonged fatigue had persistent fatigue lasting longer than six months (Bates, 1993). A surprisingly small number of these patients had their fatigue attributed to an obvious medical disorder, less than 30%.

A random survey in Wichita, Kansas estimated that 2% of the population fit the criteria for fibromyalgia, with 3.4% of women and 0.5% of men affected. The prevalence seemed to increase somewhat with age, reaching more than 7.0% in females between the ages of 60 and 79 (Wolfe, 1995). Other studies have suggested even higher rates of affliction, between 2.1 and 5.7%, and fibromyalgia typically accounts for up to 20% of patients seen by rheumatology subspecialists. Chronic fatigue syndrome itself is somewhat less prevalent, affecting 0.6% to 1.5% of the population if the strict definition outlined by the Center for Disease Control is used.

The impact of Somatoneural Dysfunction is staggering. Fibromyalgia patients referred to rheumatology specialty centers averaged 10 outpatient medical visits and used an average of 5.4 medications per year. They were hospitalized at least once every three years. This all resulted in a cost of over $2000 per patient per year (Wolfe, 1997). Patients diagnosed with chronic fatigue syndrome may rack up as much as $10,000 per year in health related costs. For Somatoneural Dysfunction on the whole, let us assume conservatively that 5% of the population is affected in a given year and the average health care cost per person is $3000. This amounts to a staggering amount somewhere in excess of thirty billion dollars per year in the United States alone. Yes, that is billion. I checked the number of zeros twice.

If you also add the lost productivity from time off from work due to the effects of Somatoneural Dysfunction, the financial impact on our society may be greater than any other single medical disorder. However, because the medical profession has in the past known so little about the problem and often passed it off as due to stress or psychosomatic illness, very little has been done to address it. The National Institute of Health spent only about $40 million dollars on research into fibromyalgia, chronic fatigue syndrome, and other related ailments in the last ten years. This is less than $1/10^{th}$ of the money spent on other chronic illnesses of much less impact.

So, if 24% of the population has unexplained chronic fatigue and only 3-5% or so have fibromyalgia or chronic fatigue syndrome, what about everybody else? Ahh, a very good question, I'm glad you asked. As you may recall from just a few sentences above, I think that these folks have Somatoneural Dysfunction. That is what the next few hundred pages will attempt to explain. This means that fibromyalgia and chronic fatigue syndromes are specific subtypes of SND, although not everyone with SND has fibromyalgia or chronic fatigue syndrome. Got it? Then read on…

The History

In 1988, the Center for Disease Control proposed criteria for the diagnosis of chronic fatigue syndrome. Around the same time, the American College of Rheumatism sought to develop criteria that defined fibromyalgia. The remainder of the 20-40 million Americans who suffer from time to time with chronic idiopathic fatigue have never been diagnosed or told why they have the problems that they do. I have written this book to describe a common pathology that links these two major disorders and encompasses the rest of these patients who don't fall nicely into any one category.

Many people assume that these problems developed when they gained popular attention in the late 1980s, but individual cases and even widespread "epidemics" have been occurring for centuries. They did not catch the public eye or the interest of the medical communities in these earliest years for the following obvious reasons:

1) With thousands dying from smallpox, tuberculosis, famine, and war, no one had any time to address something as mundane as chronic fatigue, and

2) The average life expectancy just was not long enough for these chronic conditions to manifest.

Actually, the first documented occurrences of what was probably chronic fatigue syndrome occurred aboard His Brittanic Majesty's Sloop, *Resolution* among the crew of Captain James Cook during his voyages in the South Seas. The journals of crewman Johann Reinhold Forster contain details of an ailment that sounds suspiciously like chronic fatigue syndrome and may be similar to symptoms experienced by patients in the year 2001 in America.

Reinhold noted these symptoms about a month after setting sail from New Zealand. He reported feeling "poor and weak" and was unable to "recover strength and vigor" after minor exertion. He wrote,

> "I have not yet gathered all my strength from
> my rheumatism and weakness in January, for
> I could hardly go on…I felt myself quite spent…
> I could hardly read or write…a great weakness in
> my eyes…Am brought very low…despair is
> visibly painted on all faces."

He further noted headaches, sore throat, swollen glands, "flying rheumatic pains in my limbs", and inability to sleep. Dozens of other crew members were similarly afflicted (St. George, 1996 and Hoare, 1982).

In general the crew remained in good physical health and spirits throughout their journey, making it unlikely that infectious illness or depression were responsible for these symptoms. They were a seasoned crew used to the rigors of such long trips. Similarly, it was too soon during the voyage to allow that vitamin deficiencies were the cause of the disorder, and no mention was ever made of allergic or toxic effects during the trip.

Somatoneural Dysfunction undoubtedly has been around even longer, dating back to biblical times and probably farther (Smythe, 1989). A passage in the Book of Psalms reads:

> Have mercy on me O Lord, for I am weak:
> O Lord heal me: for my bones are vexed, but
> thou O Lord, how long…I am weary with
> my groaning; all the night I make my bed to
> swim; I water my couch with tears.
>
> Psalm 6:2-6

Job spoke of insomnia, pains in his bones and joints, and profound fatigue even before he was tested by the devil. Sometimes, sufferers of SND may feel that they are being made to suffer by a higher power too. Fortunately, plague and locusts are not part of the syndrome. Famous historical figures such as Elizabeth Barrett Browning, Charles Darwin, and Florence Nightingale were afflicted with lifelong fatigue, though they were otherwise physically and psychologically healthy and lived to ripe old ages (Kim, 1994).

Sir Richard Manningham, in 1750, spoke of febricula ("little fever"), which was described as a "listlessness, with great lassitude and weariness all over the body...with little flying pains". He observed that the condition was worsened by emotional stress.

The late nineteenth century was a time of explosive advances in medical science. For the first time, physicians and scientists began to attempt to analyze and understand disease processes, and numerous infectious diseases and systemic ailments were described. In Germany, Virchow, Muller, and their students proposed the idea that micro-organisms were responsible for infectious disease. In France, Brown-Sequard founded endocrinology and spoke of hormones secreted in one part of the body and causing an effect on other parts. The great clinicians of Europe, Graves, Stokes, Addison, and Hodgkin developed and refined the physical examination of the patient. In Britain, the surgeons Bell and Paget made dramatic advances, assisted by the discoveries of nitrous oxide and ether for anesthesia. And in America, William Osler developed the system of medical analysis and education that allowed for the progress of today's medical schools and teaching hospitals.

Despite all these dramatic advances, the exploration of the cause and treatment of fatigue and similar symptoms were left somewhat behind. It is easy to see that, when faced by the great mysteries of tuberculosis, polio, diabetes, and heart disease, the doctors and researchers of the time had their collective hands quite full. Yet, descriptions of "neurasthenia" and "fibrositis" began to creep into the medical literature as their impact on society became more widely recognized. The problem was that these early medical explorers had no idea what they were doing and sometimes made erroneous conclusions that took decades to undo. Unfortunately, a majority of physicians practicing today has not advanced beyond the nineteenth century in their understanding of chronic fatigue and SND.

The great American neurologist George Beard, MD brought out the concept of neurasthenia or nervous exhaustion with his writings. He characterized patients with profound physical and mental fatigue, nervous dyspepsia, changes in mood, and protracted post-exertional fatigue (Beard, 1962). Most practitioners of the time regarded neurasthenia as predominantly a disorder of women and hard-working professionals (Abbey, 1991). I suspect that men and the lower classes of the nineteenth century had no time to become fatigued, instead fending off infection, nutritional deficiency, and trauma. With the medical advances and improvements in living conditions today, we've realized that SND knows no economic, racial, or gender boundaries.

Beard envisioned the nervous system as a delicately balanced control center for mental and physical functioning. He theorized that steam power, the telegraph, newspapers, and similar technologies were depleting the body's nervous energy. He thought this particularly evident in women, who were, of course, the weaker gender and even more delicately balanced and susceptible to perturbation. When these stressors disrupted the body's internal balance, important bodily systems such as the brain, digestive tract, and reproductive system would be affected.

Please note, ladies, that Old Dr.Beard said this and not me!

The concept of neurasthenia was a difficult one to understand all those decades ago, limited by lack of objective findings or standardized criteria for diagnosis. It remained a diagnosis of exclusion and given its broad and vague spectrum of symptoms, nearly any disorder could be characterized as "neurasthenic". It became common practice to label any patient that a physician could not accurately diagnose as having neurasthenia. Unfortunately, physicians at the turn of the century did not have the knowledge to adequately diagnose the majority of their patients. Neurasthenia thus became a dumping ground for all sorts of problems (Henderson, 1994). If you walked into a nine-teenth-century medical office with hypothyroidism, depression, diabetes, or leukemia, you would most likely be told you had neurasthenia, and not to worry so much. Fortunately, the doctors of the 21st century do a better job, albeit sometimes not much better…

Neurasthenia was then adopted by psychiatry and the field of psycho-somatic medicine was born. Its boundaries were blurred into depression, hypochondriasis, hysteria, and a multitude of other psychiatric illnesses. Medical doctors lost interest and psychiatrists attempted to explain the disorder in terms of Freudian theory and psychological disturbance for the next hundred or so years.

Beard, however, remained convinced that, despite a lack of observable physical findings, the disease was not psychological. He recognized cor-rectly that future advances in diagnostic techniques and knowledge of physiology and human function would result in proof that a somatic process was indeed responsible. He did not, however, suspect that it would take nearly a century for this to occur.

In Britain, the famous clinician William Richard Gowers coined the term "fibrositis" to explain the exquisite trigger point tenderness he found in some patients afflicted with rheumatism. He assumed that this disorder was similar to what would become known as rheumatoid arthritis, but where as the bones and joints in RA were obviously inflamed and fre-quently deformed, those in rheumatism were unremarkable to clinical and pathological examination (Wallace, 1984).

Gowers brought forth the concept of referred pain and advanced the notion that pain was governed by the central nervous system. He described a hypersensitivity of muscles, bones, and joints and believed it due to the action at nerve endings supplying the painful areas. He also believed that psychological factors, exhaustion, and sleep deprivation could contribute to the amplification of pain perception. He was really the first to accurately describe tender points, those painful, aching spots that plague many victims of Somatoneural Dysfunction.

> "It may or may not right to regard this persistent hyper-
> sensitiveness after strain as inflammatory.
> We cannot indeed distinguish it from inflammation,
> and yet we need much more pathological study before
> we can confidently assert its nature… These firm
> fibrous structures consist of compact supporting tissue
> and of nerves and nerve endings. The enduring
> sensitiveness after injury is certain evidence of changes
> in the latter."

In fact, the ideas proposed by Gowers took decades to prove, and the pain "hyperresponsiveness" in fibromyalgia and related SND states was not accepted as fact until the last few years, and then not by everyone in the medical field.

One of the problems facing early researchers in chronic fatigue syndrome was that cases tended to cluster together. Different groups of people began to experience similar symptoms beginning around the 1930s and continued to occur sporadically until a better understanding of the disorder came about in the late 1980s. These clusters of patients were viewed as either having an infectious illness or some form of mass hysteria. Infectious disease specialists studied these clusters in great detail in an attempt to find a causative microorganism. This fruitless effort continued for nearly sixty years and implicated various innocent bacteria, viruses, protozoa, and fungi. It is unfortunate and ironic that such an effort was wasted looking for something that isn't there. If you look at the symptoms of low-grade fever, swollen glands, and malaise, and the clustering of cases, however, it is easy to see why an infection was assumed to be responsible.

The search for an elusive infectious agent led to the coining of phrases such as "epidemic neuromyasthenia", "benign myalgic encephalomyelitis", "chronic mononucleosis-like syndrome", "post-viral fatigue syndrome" and "epidemic poliomyelitis-like illness". Generally, medical researchers give the longest names to syndromes that they don't understand.

The first well-documented cluster of cases in the United States occurred in Los Angeles in 1934. A widespread polio epidemic occurred in California in 1934 and many of the sickest patients were cared for at the Los Angeles County General Hospital in the spring of that year. Starting around May, workers at the hospital began experiencing symptoms of muscle tenderness and sensitivity, insomnia, emotional upset, paresthesias, sensory disturbances, localized muscle weakness, and neck and back stiffness (Shelokov, 1957). A total of 210 people, mostly women, and mostly nurses and student nurses were affected.

Despite intensive investigation for polio and other infections, no cause was ever found. Many of the patients were hospitalized even though they never had a fever or other sign of systemic illness. There were no deaths, but a majority were unable to work; 54% were still absent from duty six months later. Their symptoms appeared to be exacerbated by cold weather and the onset of their menstrual cycle, common findings in other similar outbreaks and in SND sufferers today. A few of the patients were left with lasting symptoms, some as long as 30 years (Henderson, 1994).

Over the next twenty or so years, several more outbreaks of a similar disorder were noted during polio epidemics in locations as diverse as Iceland (1948), Durban, South Africa (1955), London (1955) and Coventry (1953), England, Adelaide, Australia (1949), Copenhagen, Denmark (1952), Washington, DC (1953), and New York City (1952). Patients in each outbreak experienced easy fatigue with exertion, chronic dull headaches, and diffuse muscle aches. Nearly all of them had sleep disturbances, self-reported (though rarely documented) fevers, and concentration problems.

The Washington, D.C. outbreak affected 29 of 41 female student nurses at a community hospital that cared for many polio patients. Only 1 of 19 male physicians and 1 of 72 hospital patients were also affected.

Spinal taps, blood cultures, and urine samples were all tested for infectious organisms without any positive findings. Upon follow-up four years later, many still had significant disability and 85% suffered from muscle stiffness, fatigue, tender points, and weakness made worse by cold weather, menstrual periods, and physical exertion (Henderson, 1994).

The Iceland outbreak struck 465 people in the rural village of Akureyi, most of those afflicted were boarders at a public high school, many under the age of 21 and about 37% male. They seemed to suffer from a variety of neurologic and psychologic complaints, including muscle weakness, nervousness, sleeplessness, and memory loss. Six years later, many still suffered extreme fatigue and tiredness despite their youth and apparent good health. Some were unable to keep physically active and showed signs of muscle atrophy from disuse (Sigurdsson, 1950).

The other outbreaks followed similar courses, mostly striking young adults in nursing and closely associated fields. In London, over 200 patients were hospitalized and suffered from "Extreme fatigue…making the rehabilitation period extremely long and tedious." Several months later, many patients "with the best will in the world were often only able to work for four hours a day" (McEvedy, 1970).

In Florida, during the mid-1950s, several outbreaks began to occur outside of hospitals and clinics and in patients outside of the medical professions. Drs. James Bond (the Florida epidemiologist and not the secret agent) and Harold Wolff (professor of neurology at Cornell Medical School) investigated the "epidemic" in Leon County, Florida, near Tallahassee. They documented 460 cases, a very large number in a county of only 60,000 population total. Seventy percent were women with 4% of all the females in the county between the ages of 25-34 affected. Most, but not all, of the patients had contact with someone previously ill, and the vast majority were white (Wallace, 1984)

Once again, extensive testing failed to turn up a viral or other infectious cause. Despite that, however, investigators remained convinced that such an agent must be responsible. They concluded that the epidemic was caused by an unknown virus spread from person-to-person with the range of symptoms "modified by the physiological or serological differences that exist between youth and middle age, male and female, negro and white, and perhaps married and unmarried" (Wallace, 1984).

This was interesting commentary indeed. This postulates that there could be a virus that affects people depending on differences such as marital status. Husbands bitten by "the golfing bug" and wives with "shopping flu" notwithstanding, there are not any viral agents that are smart enough to make this distinction. Furthermore, infections, unlike systemic or genetic illnesses, do not generally affect a single race, gender, or age. Certainly, some illnesses manifest with different severity in patients of different susceptibilities based on overall health and hygiene, but these cases were healthy young adults being affected. One would surmise that infections would hit the elderly and debilitated more readily, but these groups were actually spared.

Interestingly, again, Leon County was the site of an aggressive awareness and fund-raising campaign by the March of Dimes in support of victims with polio. Could such an epidemic stem from a type of mass hypochondriasis or hysteria? Certainly, sufferers of SND have been told that by doctors for years, and have likely considered it themselves. Throughout history, however, patients with seemingly unexplainable symptoms and syndromes have been thought to have psychological disturbances, only to find a true medical disease state after years of searching.

The next year, in Punta Gorda, Florida, another cluster of cases (numbering about one hundred) occurred over a three-month period. Dr. David Poskanzer, a neurologist and epidemiologist assigned by the CDC to investigate the case, reported patients with disturbances in memory and mentation, muscle weakness and tenderness, menstrual irregularities, and a whole host of neurologic signs and symptoms, most of which made little neuroanatomic sense. He presented his findings to a panel of experts at the CDC's Epidemic Intelligence Service and was called "incoherent", "inexperienced", and generally derided for his "epidemic", which most on the panel thought sounded like widespread neurotic behavior (Briggs, 1994).

Nonetheless, perhaps spurred as much by the desire to bask in the Florida sunshine as analytic curiosity, a group of scientists returned to the site for further investigation. Poskanzer was accompanied by Dr. Charles Kunkle, professor of neurology at Duke, Dr. Sy Kalter, head of virology at the CDC, and Dr. D.A. Henderson (perhaps the founding father of chronic fatigue syndrome and SND). Henderson, a brilliant epidemiologist, physician, and virologist, would much later go on to become Assistant Secretary for Health and Human Services (Briggs, 1994).

This distinguished group, however, found itself no more able than Poskanzer alone to come up with an adequate explanation for the case. They selected a group of patients and performed detailed clinical and laboratory examinations. The examinations were repeated 5 and 12 months later, and still failed to determine any related cause. Clinically, they found patients with muscle weakness, but normal tone, bulk, and reflexes. They encountered lymph node swellings that appeared and disappeared at random. They noted patchy areas of increased sensitivity to pain and pressure and mapped them out on patients' skin, only to find completely different areas affected the next day (Briggs, 1994).

The group still suspected a viral cause, suggesting that it resulted in dysfunction of the autonomic nervous system. Actually, the autonomic nervous system, which is responsible for regulatory and "emergency" functioning of the other bodily systems, is indeed intimately involved in Somatoneural Dysfunction. Unfortunately, investigators focused on the infectious hypotheses for decades instead. Probably, this occurred from a practical sense rather than scientific error. During that time period, remarkable advances in the ability to culture, identify, and analyze microorganisms was growing exponentially, culminating with the invention of the electron microscope in the 1930s. Virology was thus the new and extremely fascinating science of the time and attempts were made wherever possible to discover and characterize new viruses. It was in this veritable virologic "feeding frenzy" that the true nature of SND was over-looked.

On the other hand, psychiatry was a growing science as well. The notion that the brain and central nervous system influenced medical illness and bodily functions was the great breakthrough of the science of neurology. Psychiatry had just begun to catch up in the 1920s and 1930s, implying that mood, emotions, and thought processes could also impact on health and well-being. This effort blended with traditional medicine in the field of psychosomatics, which remained a poorly understood and derided field until the last two decades or so.

McEvedy and Beard published two articles, in the *British Medical Journal* in 1970, which analyzed the 1955 outbreak at Royal Free Hospital in London. They used the term benign myalgic encephalomyelitis, but concluded that the patients all suffered from hysteria and suggested alternatively that the disorder be called "myalgia nervosa". They observed that the majority of patients were female (attributing again the supposed susceptibility of women to hysteria and neurosis), had no significant laboratory abnormalities, and little or no signs of systemic illness such as fever (McEvedy, 1970).

Interestingly, other researchers found this outbreak to be the one with cases that had the most physical abnormalities. These patients suffered "severe and widespread involvement of the central nervous system", abnormalities in muscle tone and reflexes, cranial nerve signs, nystagmus, muscle spasm, "a peculiar jerking...on voluntary movement", objective sensory deficits on neurologic exam, and even paralysis (Briggs, 1994). This hardly sounds like something hysterical or intentional.

Why did these investigators come to the conclusion that the disorder was purely psychological? Possibly, some of the other symptoms of the patients at Royal Free Hospital led them in this direction. Patients suffered from complaints of "hypersomnia, of nightmares, and of panic states, and sometimes uncontrolled weeping" in addition to their fatigue, muscle aches, and headaches. What McEvedy, Beard, and others did not fully grasp at the time is that no disease is entirely psychological or physical, but rather a blending of both, each with profound influences on one another.

Imagine suffering from an illness that makes you feel terrible, unable to work or care for your family, have headaches and muscle aches all the time, and strange nervous system defects. Of course, many of you readers who live with Somatoneural Dysfunction can imagine this quite well. Now imagine that no one has any idea why this is happening to you and that virologists from the Center for Disease Control have descended upon your town in search of the "new virus" that you have. Would you have nightmares? Sleep disturbances? Might you suffer from depression and panic? I certainly would, and I see my patients fifty years later go through the same types of things.

Unfortunately, instead of recognizing that psychological factors contribute strongly to the overall picture of SND and investigating this link, many researchers simply dismissed the disorder as "being all in your head".

Thus, we had two groups of scientists interested in SND back in the middle of the century; one investigating it as an infection, the other as a psychological disorder. As we shall discuss in much of the rest of this book, both the immune system and the psyche are important in the etiology and understanding of SND, but neither alone is at the root of the problem. In fact, they are closely connected, a point that was not really established until 1982 in Rochester, New York.

The investigators then established criteria for investigating further outbreaks, thinking still that an infection was responsible, but that they had simply missed it in the previous outbreaks. A period of five years went by with only a sporadic case here and there. However, the major outbreaks of the next twenty years nicely illustrated the great diversity of SND.

Twenty-six nuns in a convent in upstate New York came down with an illness characterized by abnormal sensory findings, weakness, stomach upset, and extreme fatigue worsened by physical or mental activity and the onset of their menstrual cycles. In addition, "most patients felt tense, nervous, or unusually depressed…many had to give up their studies and classes because they 'simply couldn't think' " (Albrecht, 1964). This time, the CDC scientists were there to take samples not only from the patients but their surroundings as well, thinking perhaps that contaminated food, water, or air was involved. Again they found nothing, despite nearly a year of intensive research and follow-up. Similar investigations of outbreaks in Rockville, Maryland and Ridgefield, Connecticut reached similar inconclusions.

The convent outbreak occurred without relation to polio epidemics, in fact, coming nearly ten years after the advent of the polio vaccine when cases had dwindled to rare. Therefore, it was unlikely that any physiologic (or even psychosomatic) relation to polio had occurred. In addition, it seemed implausible that the nuns had all developed hysteria, anxiety disorder, or depression together at roughly the same time.

Other cases began to occur in diverse areas around the world. In West Otago, New Zealand, researchers evaluated 28 cases among patients of Maori heritage and found symptoms of prolonged fatigue, transient diarrhea, and chronic upper respiratory symptoms. Upon follow-up ten years later, 10 of the patients fit the standard definition of chronic fatigue syndrome, while another 11 were classified as having chronic idiopathic fatigue. The remaining seven continued to be undiagnosed. Most were able to return to their prior level of functioning, but many had persistent symptoms that necessitated significant lifestyle and work changes (Levine, 1997).

Typically, adults of young and middle age are most often stricken with Somatoneural Dysfunction. However, no age is truly spared, even children. Between 1984 and 1987, 21 cases occurring in children between the ages of 6 and 17 were noted in Yates, New York, a rural community of only 2,371 residents. Thirty-eight percent of the children experienced paresthesias, two-thirds had memory loss and poor concentration, and another 24% suffered speech disturbances (Bell, 1991).

Overall, these clusters illustrate several points. Patients who have Somatoneural Dysfunction suffer an extremely variable presentation and course of illness. They come in all ages, both genders, varied ethnic backgrounds, and diverse socioeconomic status. SND has features of illness that spans all human organ systems, but mainly involves the central nervous system, musculoskeletal system, and immune system. Psychological factors play an important role in defining, understanding, and treating the syndrome.

So far, I have implied that SND is neither an infectious process, nor a psychological one. If that is the case, you, the astute reader may ask, why did these early cases seem to occur in clusters? To answer that, we must understand both human nature and the limitations of the medical profession at the times of the "epidemics".

The simplest explanation stems from the fact that SND does not typically elicit dramatic physical signs or symptoms. Patients may feel diffuse muscle aches, headaches, and fatigue as the primary components. None of these symptoms are usually alarming or severe enough to seek medical attention. Patients assume that their symptoms will improve with time and that they are suffering from typical every-day aches and pains of human life. It is not until the symptoms persist for unusually long periods of time, weeks, months, or even years, that patients finally consider that they may have a medical illness.

Furthermore, during the middle part of the century, nothing was known about SND, so it would be quite difficult for patients to realize they had it on their own. Once cases begin to appear, however, others felt more legitimized in reporting their own condition. Even now, with the wealth of medical information and communication available to patients, I see people every week who have SND and don't realize it. I then read them the list of signs and symptoms or perhaps a patient case until they realize, "My goodness, that sounds exactly like me". Patients decades ago were no different.

In fact, rather than reporting their illness, many patients tried to mask their symptoms or "tough it out". Many felt they would be viewed as weak, silly, or even crazy if they complained of their problem. This was particularly true in cases where a neuropsychological component was prominent. Symptoms such as poor concentration, nervousness, memory loss, and depression are often dismissed as psychosomatic today, let alone fifty years ago.

As we begin to understand the impact that stress has on the immune and central nervous systems, we can also see why these clusters tended to occur in caregivers of patients afflicted with contagious diseases. These caregivers lived in constant fear of contracting life-threatening diseases from the patients they cared for. Add the hectic workload of caregivers during these epidemics, and it becomes easier to see their susceptibility to illness.

So while investigators labored fruitlessly in search of new viruses in Punta Gorda, West Otago, Los Angelas, and elsewhere, I am certain that millions of others went about their daily lives as best they could, suffering from the same things as those in the "epidemic". Now, in the new millennium, the medical profession must not only strive to diagnose and treat the patients who appear in our clinics and offices, but to inform and educate the population as a whole, so that there is a greater understanding of this common and costly disorder. Only with education and understanding can we undertake the challenge of treatment and cure.

Chapter 2:
The Symptoms and Signs of Somatoneural Dysfunction

To understand what this disorder is, where it came from, and how to treat it, there has to be a concept of the physiological basis and influencing factors. I lecture frequently to medical students and residents an am surprised at how little they know about why certain symptoms occur. They know, for example, that diabetes mellitus stems from a lack of insulin secretion from the pancreas. When I ask them, however, why diabetic patients are hungry and thisty all the time, why they get headaches and dizziness when their sugar goes too low, or how high levels of sugar damage the eyes, kidneys, and heart, they are often at a loss for an explanation.

Therefore I am going to use the next few chapters to explain, in a simple and concise way, what is going wrong in Somatoneural Dysfunction and why some of the symptoms occur. This chapter will discuss how some of the processes that become dysfunctional in SND work when they are going right. I promise you that most of this is not really all that complicated, despite the fact that the medical profession sometimes likes to try and keep patients in the dark. One of the most frequent and unfortunate mistakes physicians make when dealing with their patients is assuming that they are not able to understand the complex issues of medical science and not explaining things properly to them. I, on the other hand, will assume that my readers are brilliant. You have, after all, purchased this book...

The criteria set forth in later chapters may help you understand the specific syndromes of fibromyalgia and chronic fatigue syndrome, but it is my belief that these disorders represent a minority subset of all patients with Somatoneural Dysfunction. Keep this in mind as you read the following section, noting that a particular patient may have any combination of these symptoms and to a highly variable degree of severity.

Fatigue

Well now, this is certainly a good place to start. If you don't have fatigue, congratulations, you probably don't have Somatoneural Dys-function. Fatigue is the hallmark of SND, the only single factor that is invariably present. Patients with SND are tired, fatigued, exhausted, bushed, weary, and generally pooped out.

Of course, everyone is fatigued sometime or other, but the fatigue prevalent in SND is different from this normal fatigue in two ways. It is more severe and difficult to overcome, interfering in one's everyday life and making the simplest activities difficult. It is also more prolonged; most definitions require six months or more of fatigue to be labeled as abnormal. Certainly SND results in fatigue that is more severe and longlasting than is typical, but a key that I look for is whether or not this fatigue results in a decreased level of functioning.

When a patient explains to me that they are feeling too tired to go to work, do chores around the house, or go out to a movie there is probably a problem. The only way this would not be abnormal is if the patient never went to work, did chores around the house, or went out to a movie. This is another situation entirely, most often seen in teenagers and some husbands I know. More commonly, patient with SND are still able to work, do chores, and go out, but they often do so at a lower level of efficiency and it may take a great deal of effort to overcome their fatigue. They have to constantly push themselves. Somatoneural Dysfunction results in a change from a previous level of functioning that is apparent to the patient and most likely to those around them.

Abnormal fatigue as defined in the Center for Disease Control's criteria for the diagnosis of chronic fatigue syndrome is:

> "Clinically evaluated, unexplained, persistent or
> relapsing fatigue that is of new or definite onset;
> is not the result of ongoing exertion; is not substantially
> alleviated by rest; and results in substantial reduction in pre-
> vious levels of occupational, educational, social, or
> personal activities (CDC Guidelines)."

This brief statement illustrates several important factors in the fatigue associated with SND. Many patients can pinpoint the start of their symptoms of fatigue to a specific time or event. This is in contrast to the fatigue that often accompanies depression or chronic medical illnesses, which is typically diffuse in origin and more vague in nature. Sometimes, the abruptness of onset of the fatigue in SND initiates a "wild goose chase" to determine a different medical cause.

Mrs. S could pinpoint the start of her SND related fatigue. One day she opened her refrigerator door and felt "a cold wind come upon" her. From that day on she suffered from tremendous fatigue and joint aches from SND, not cold winds or refrigerators

Normally, fatigue is accompanied by a feeling of weakness, which occurs as a result of a series of biochemical and physiologic changes in muscles and a reduced capacity to generate force. Continuous muscular exertion leads to depletion of adenosine triphosphate (ATP). This biochemical can be viewed as the energy current of the human body. Often

when I speak of this "energy", my patients look at me skeptically, thinking
I have lapsed into the metaphysical realm and
expect me to read their palms or bring out
some Tarot cards. Yet, ATP really does exist
and is involved in thousands of chemical reactions that are necessary each time we perform
any type of physical activity.

If activity is continued beyond the point
where ATP is depleted, the body's backup system of anaerobic metabolism kicks in. This
process generates more ATP by breaking
down glycogen, which is stored in muscle and
fat. Once this supply of ATP is used up as

Muscle Activity
↓
Depletion of ATP
↓
Depletion of glycogen
↓
Use of fatty acids
↓
Accumulation of lactate
↓
Fatigue

well, muscular activity cannot continue at peak efficiency, resulting in
fatigue and weakness. Even then, the body has an emergency backup system that allows fatty acids to be converted into energy. Use of this system,
however, causes problems later as lactic acid (lactate) accumulates. This
reduces muscle contraction and delays the recovery of muscle strength
(Kandel & Schwartz, 2000). When this fatigued state is reached, two
important things happen: 1) there is a subjective feeling of tiredness and
lack of energy, and 2) a decreased capacity for work and productivity
occurs.

It is this lack of energy leads to what I call the "vicious cycle" of
Somatoneural Dysfunction. Simply stated, patients who are tired all the
time have difficulty engaging in physical activity. Normally, rest replen-
ishes the body's supply of ATP energy and the feeling of tiredness is allevi-
ated. In those with SND, however, this system of re-energizing is defective
and chronic, enabling longlasting fatigue to set in. This is much like being
trapped in a tunnel cave in, where the more dirt you dig out the more falls
into the tunnel, making escape harder and harder. Thus, patients with
SND find themselves completely exhausted after physical or mental exertion, making them less and less likely to undertake such efforts in the

future. I have seen this phenomenon time and time again lead to true weakness and deconditioning, which further complicates the picture.

It is partly this decreased productivity and capacity for work that leads to some of the striking psychological aspects of SND. A patient in a persistently fatigued state has an impaired ability to make sound judgements and decisions. This in turn creates feelings of inadequacy and low self-esteem, which may ultimately lead to anxiety and depression. Difficulties and conflicts at work may lead to increased stress, which exacerbates fatigue and SND in general. Furthermore, the natural response to stress is avoidance, which can result not only in lateness or absence from work, but poor overall work performance. Similarly, difficulties with family and friends in social situations can lead to avoidance and withdrawal from important social support systems.

As I have mentioned, fatigue is present in all types of Somatoneural Dysfunction. It is also seen in virtually every other chronic medical problem, as a side effect of many medications, as a component of many primary psychiatric illnesses, and as an element of the everyday lives of hardworking people throughout the world. It is this ubiquity that has made fatigue syndromes difficult to diagnose and differentiate.

Pain

> **Pain**, n. an uncomfortable frame of mind
> that may have a physical basis in something
> that is being done to the body, or may be
> purely mental, caused by the good fortune of
> another (Bierce, 1856).

Pain has been called, "nature's earliest sign of morbidity". It is an integral part of the body's built-in natural defense mechanisms, the one that says, "hey, take your hand off of that hot stove, you idiot, before you burn your hand off". Pain is not very tactful. Consequently, pain protects us from injuring ourselves by avoiding painful stimuli. It also is a symptom of many (if not most) internal medical problems and prompts us to seek medical help. There are actually two different types of pain, acute and chronic, which are two separate, but interrelated systems present in the brain and spinal cord. Pain is most prominent in patients with the fibromyalgia type of SND, but may contribute markedly to other types as well.

From Here to There

Probably the most difficult aspect of understanding pain is figuring out how painful information gets from the site of pain to the brain where the information is processed. There are basically three parts of the pain-response system: the receptor, the transmitter, and the receiver.

The receptors are usually nerve endings in the area of the body where pain is first sensed, either on or near the skin or within the deep structures of the body. Skin pain is usually the type brought about by some trauma (burning, pricking, poking, and so on) and is comprised of two components called the "double response of Lewis". The first component is the initial pain of traumatic contact. This information is carried on large, fast transmitting nerve fibers called A-δ. This is followed by a stinging or burning pain transmitted across a different set of nerve fibers that are smaller and slower, referred to as C fibers. This type of pain is more diffuse and enduring (Harrison, 2000).

Deep pain from internal organs or musculoskeletal structures is caused by stretch or spasm. If you poke your gallbladder with a pin (although I don't recommend you try this at home), it doesn't hurt; there are no "skin" receptors there to carry painful information. If, however, the gallbladder stretches and distends, due, say, to a gallstone blocking the exit duct, it can double you over and send you rushing to the nearest emergency room. Deep pain can either be acute (a sharp, knife-like pain from stretch or a crampy type of pain from spasm) or chronic (an inflammatory type of pain secondary to the initial insult).

Once pain is sensed at the nerve ending, the information is transmitted across the nerve fiber to neurons in an area of the spinal cord called the dorsal horn. Many of the fibers travel through the spinal cord in a bundle called Lissauer's tract before they connect at the spinal cord relay station of the dorsal horn. Each sensory unit has a unique localization from the nerve ending through the spinal cord to the brain. For

> Step 1: pain information travels from the nerve ending to the dorsal horn of the spinal cord via Lissauer's tract.

skin pain, these units can be mapped out in discrete areas called dermatomes (Figure 1).

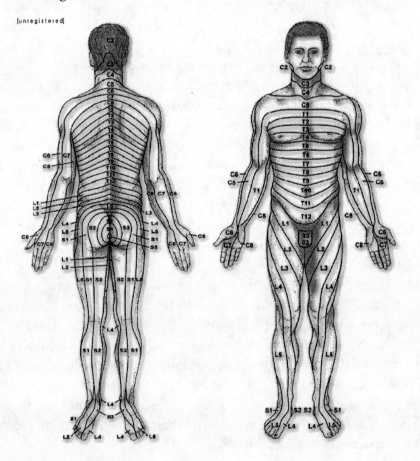

[unregistered]

Each dermatome on the skin can be traced back to a specific level of the spinal cord. Thus, if you hit the tip of your middle finger with a hammer, the painful information is carried to nerve cells that enter the spinal cord at the level of the 7th cervical vertebra (C7). Interestingly, this pathway can be a two-way street. If, for example, you have a ruptured disk that causes pressure to be exerted on the C7 nerve root, you probably will have pain (or numbness and tingling) in the tip of your middle finger.

The localization of deep pain from internal organs and musculo-skeletal structures is a bit more complicated. Here the pain is referred to the skin innervated by the same spinal segment and not the skin overlying the painful structure. This may be quite far away from the source of pain and thus can be somewhat misleading. The pain of a stomach ulcer or inflammation of the pancreas may be felt in the back, not the front, while pain from a heart attack may refer to the jaw or down the left arm. Further complicating matters is the fact that visceral pain (from internal organs) can also transmit its information to adjacent nerve roots, making it diffuse and difficult to pinpoint.

> Step 2: information is relayed up the spinal cord by the spinaothalamic tract (skin pain) or the spinoreticulo-thalamic tract (deep pain).

From the dorsal horn, the pain impulse is relayed up the spinal cord to the brain. Most of the pain from the skin is carried in the spinothalamic tract, which ends in the thalamus, one of the main relay centers of the brain. Deep pain is carried predominantly on the spinoreticulothalamic tract, a bundle of fibers that projects to the reticular nucleus in the midbrain as well as to the thalamus. This tract is more diffuse and subject to influences at a number of sites along the way, such as descending inhibitory connections from the raphe nucleus. This helps to control the strength and extent of the pain.

The thalamus performs an extremely complex task of organizing incoming information about painful stimuli and projecting it on to different areas of higher function in the brain for final processing and interpretation.

One group of thalamic neurons sends projections to the primary sensory cortex, which is involved in discrimination of pain and other sensory information. This allows pain to be localized to a certain point on the body, such that if you close your left thumb in the waffle iron, you don't pull away your right foot. Another

> Step 3: information is relayed up to the cerebral cortex for interpretation

group of neurons transmits to the hypothalamus and mediates the autonomic nervous system response to pain, such as sweating, increased heart rate and blood pressure, and the sick feeling of nausea that occurs when a baseball player takes a line drive in the you-know-where. Still another area of the thalamus projects its information to the limbic system where the emotional response to pain occurs.

All three of these higher brain structures are therefore involved in the final processing and interpretation of pain. Together, they serve two main functions in response to a painful event. They mobilize the body's defense mechanisms to avoid painful stimuli and to trigger the immune system and musculoskeletal system to suppress or eliminate the inciting event. Unfortunately, sometimes these systems cause further discomfort by inducing spasm or inflammation in the process of eliminating the painful stimuli. Spasm of smooth or skeletal muscle is designed to get rid of the noxious factor that is causing the problem, while inflammation is necessary to repair tissue injury and dilute offending toxins. Even more importantly, the brain acts to directly modulate and lessen pain in a number of different ways through descending pathways.

The first pathway of defense against pain sends commands back down to the spinal cord to decrease its intensity. The brain says, in essence, "Message received, you can stop all that throbbing now!" The area of the brain involved in this type of pain regulation is called the periaqueductal gray matter of the midbrain (an area that is in need of a new name). Another important modulating system originates in the pons, which, when activated, blocks pain receptors in the spinal cord and peripheral nerves. This system is responsible for the regulation of chronic, rather than acute types of pain (Kandel & Schwartz, 2000).

Nuts, Bolts, and Neurotransmitters

Now that we hopefully understand a little about the "hardwiring" of the nervous system with regards to pain perception, we can talk about how all this complex information is actually sent back and forth and to and fro within the nervous system. We often view the nerves in our bodies as tiny electrical cords connecting various tiny points. This is true to a certain extent, but electrical information is simply an on/off phenomenon and can't provide for interpretation. If you take an electrical cord and plug it into the wall, nothing happens. But, if you plug the other end into a television set you may see reruns of Sanford and Son™. The television set, or toaster, or waffle iron receives a message from the electrical cord to turn on and does its thing. Similarly, the nerves themselves only act to turn the receiving cells on or off.

What happens when a cell is turned on is quite amazing (even more so than the fact that reruns of Sanford and Son™ are still on television). The cell (in this case, the cell of the nervous system, the neuron) releases a chemical called a neurotransmitter or hormone that causes a specific effect on the cells to which it is connected. This takes place by means of many complex chemical reactions. There are several different types of neuro-transmitters involved in the response and modulation of pain.

The first is called Substance P, which was named by its discoverers for "pain", perhaps so they didn't forget its function. Substance P, along with glutamate and aspartate, is released at the nerve ending at the site of pain and triggers the initial response of the pain cascade. This initiates the relay process that sends information up towards the spinal cord and brain. These neurochemicals are also involved in triggering the inflammatory response at the site of pain. Though Substance P is involved in acute pain from trauma, it is even more important in chronic pain states (arthritis for example, and Somatoneural Dysfunction).

Descending pathways have three main neurotransmitters in the arsenal of defense for pain. The system of endorphins is the first line of protection. This group of chemicals, which closely resemble natural and man-made pain reliever such as morphine, act in the brain, spinal cord, and at peripheral nerves to deaden the response to pain. Norepinephrine- and acetylcholine-containing pathways extend from the pons down to the spinal cord and muscles to limit pain and allow us to override our natural protective mechanisms. This is how a football player can run down the field on a broken leg to score the winning touchdown, or how an addict on PCP (which dramatically enhances norepinephrine secretion) can take dozens of bullets and still not feel any pain. The final neurotransmitter system involves serotonin and extends from the medulla to the dorsal horn cells in the spinal cord. This system is involved in the modulation mainly of chronically painful states and is also concerned with mood and emotion.

As you can undoubtedly tell, this system is extraordinarily complex, but you only need to keep three things in mind:

1)   Pain travels from a receiver in the body through the spinal cord and to the brain.
2)   A complex system of neurotransmitters is responsible for the transmission, interpretation, and regulation of pain.
3)   The brain acts to control and modulate pain.

These are important things to remember as they are critical to theunderstanding of where things can go wrong in Somatoneural Dysfunction and what kinds of things we can do to help. But don't worry, I'll remind you a bit later.

In fibromyalgia and other types of Somatoneural Dysfunction, there are two distinct abnormalities in the pain cascade. The ascending pain pathway that brings painful information to the central nervous system is overactive and is turned on by lower levels of stimulation. A fibro patient may therefore have a painful flare of their disease with moderate exercise, a change in the weather, a minor trauma, or for no reason at all in severe cases.

The proof of this comes from some excellent studies done in fibromyalgia patients by Larson in Minnesota. Dr. Larson and co-investigators found abnormalities in the spinal fluid of fibromyalgia sufferers including elevated levels of substance P. These changes are seen at baseline and are above the levels found in other chronically painful states (Larson, 2000). There were also alterations in excitatory neurotransmitters like glutamate and aspartate that implied an abnormality in nitric oxide signaling in the CNS.

Nitric oxide is involved in a myriad of biologic activities in the human body and it is probable that abnormalities in nitric oxide generation, metabolism, and degradation are responsible, at least at the biological level, for many or all of the symptom complexes of SND. Nitric oxide cascades are certainly involved in pain perception, inflammation and the immune system, and blood vessel and muscle activity. The likely site of action of the dysfunctional nitric oxide pathways in relation to pain is the NMDA-receptor, which is discussed in further detail in the section to come on fibromyalgia.

Headache

Headaches are both very common (affecting 57% of the population every month) and prevalent in SND (roughly 90% of the cases experience some sort of headache). The development of a chronic headache syndrome may prove to be extremely difficult to treat. Overall, neurology textbooks list thirteen categories of headaches and 129 subtypes. I will discuss a few generalities about headaches and some particular aspects of headache syndromes as they relate to SND.

Patients with Somatoneural Dysfunction may suffer from three types of headache syndromes, which comprise a spectrum from migraine-type headaches, to tension-type headaches, to a chronic persistent headache syndrome. Most often we see patients that suffer from frequent tension-type headaches, punctuated by intermittent attacks of the more severe migraine-type. Too often, through inadequate treatment, lack of education about headache treatment, or stubborn symptoms, these headaches can "transform" into chronic, daily headaches, which can be quite refractory to treatment.

Migraine is a complex neuropsychologic disorder characterized by episodic and progressive forms of head pain. This pain may be accompanied by a variety of neurologic, psychologic, and autonomic disturbances. It is typically throbbing in nature, and is usually present on one side of the head only. The headache in classic migraine is preceded by an "aura", which can be any type of sensation, most often of certain sights, sounds, or smells. Migraine without an aura is sometimes called common migraine and is actually five times more common than classic migraine (Saper, 1999).

The cause of these headaches is not fully understood, but probably represents a disorder in serotonin-containing neurons in the brain. Serotonin, in addition to its many other functions, is important in the regulation and function of blood vessels in the central nervous system. Abnormal deactivation of this serotonin system in the brainstem results in spasm and inflammation of nearby blood vessels.

Tension-type headaches probably represent a variant of migraine and are generally less severe, but are more frequent and may last longer. Both types of headache may "transform" into a severe headache syndrome that occurs on a daily basis. Some patients with these transform migraines may feel as if they always have a headache. The matter is often complicated by overuse of headache medications, which results in rebound headaches.

This rebound phenomenon occurs when frequent use of pain medication leads to a change in the actual function of cells in the affected areas of the brain. These cells come to require the specific medication in order to function normally, and in essence become addicted to it. We most commonly see this with narcotic pain relievers and tranquilizers, but any pain medicine (even Tylenol™ or aspirin) can result in rebound. The only difference seems to be the quickness with which rebound and addiction occurs; narcotics can result in these changes after as little as ten days of continuous use, whereas we may not see the syndrome develop with aspirin for years.

Back Pain and Myofascial Pain

Low back pain is another extremely common affliction in this country. Four out of five people suffer from major back pain at some point in their lives, 50% each year, and 15-20% at any given moment! About 1% of the U.S. population is disabled because of back pain, which results in tremendous medical expense and loss of productivity (Rosomoff, 1999).

Obviously, there are many common causes of back pain as illustrated in table 1. With Somato-neural Dysfunction we see a specific type of back pain syndrome that has been known variously as trigger point pain tender point pain, limited or regional type fibromyalgia or more appropriately and accurately as myofascial back pain. Diagnosis of myofascial back pain relies on the exclusion of these other syndromes. Warning signs of serious causes of back pain include bowel or bladder abnormalities, true muscle weakness in the affected limbs, loss of sensation in the "saddle" area around the perineum, and loss of reflexes. Any of these warning signs, or the presence of high fever or malignancy warrants specialized testing such as MRI scanning.

Myofascial pain refers to pain emanating from the layer of fibrous connective tissue that acts as a sheath around muscles and protects and strengthens muscles, tendons, and ligaments. Pain of the myofascia can occur with stretch, spasm, or inflammation (as you could surmise from our discussion just a few pages ago). This may cause restriction of motion,tender points when the affected area is pressed, mechanical dysfunction, and fatigue (Rosomoff, 1999).

Myofascial pain syndromes of the back are divided into four types, depending on the muscle group involved. Quadratus lumborum syndrome is most common and

Table 1: Causes of Back Pain
Fracture
Muscle strain or sprain
Osteoarthritis
Rheumatoid or other inflammatory arthritides
Spondylolisthesis (slipping of the vertebrae)
Spondylolysis (bony defect in the vertebral body)
Bone spurs
Osteoporosis
Disk herniation or protrusion (sciatica)
Spinal canal stenosis (narrowing)
Paget's Disease
Arachnoiditis (inflammation between the spinal cord and connective tissue lining)
Meningitis
Osteomyelitis (infection of the bone)
Bone cancer or metastatic disease of the bone
Hemorrhage into the spinal canal
Referred pain (from chest, abdomen, or pelvis)

may manifest as pain at the iliac crest, greater trochanter, groin, or sacroiliac joint. This pain often awakens the patient in the middle of the night and is worst when climbing steps. There is also limited flexion and extension of the spine and pain when the area adjacent to the spine is pressed. Iliopsoas syndrome causes pain into the pelvis and thigh, resulting in stooped posture and abnormal rotation of the hip when walking. Gluteal and piriformis syndromes may be mistaken for sciatica and give deep pain in the buttocks or sacrum. Chapter 4 has a more detailed discussion of tender points and myofascial pain syndrome as well as a diagram of the most common locations of tender points (Figure 2).

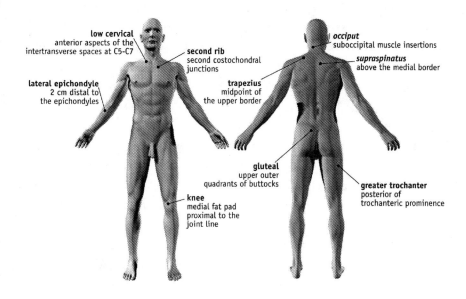

low cervical
anterior aspects of the
intertransverse spaces at C5-C7

second rib
second costochondral
junctions

lateral epichondyle
2 cm distal to
the epichondyles

trapezius
midpoint of
the upper border

occiput
suboccipital muscle insertions

supraspinatus
above the medial border

gluteal
upper outer
quadrants of buttocks

knee
medial fat pad
proximal to the
joint line

greater trochanter
posterior of
trochanteric prominence

Neuropathic Pain

Neuropathic pain is pain that stems from irritation of nerve endings, usually from pressure, injury, or inflammation. Common causes include diabetes (excess glucose can cause injury and inflammation of the nerves), viral infections such as varicella, sciatica (from nerve root compression by herniated disk material), or cancer (which causes direct nerve injury). Symptoms of neuropathy are usually described as numbing, burning, shocking, squeezing, or crawling and may be resistant to even the strongest pain relievers. These pains may be constant or result in severe intermittent flares.

The mechanism of neuropathic pain is still somewhat speculative. It appears to involve abnormal sensitization in the nerve axons (fibers) and C-conductive pathways. When these connections are damaged by any of the above causes, regeneration occurs to attempt to correct the injury. However, this process doesn't work too well after the embryonic stages of development and may either form a neuroma or remain demyelinated.

A neuroma is essentially a tangled bundle of nerve fibers with tenuous connections to surrounding neurons. These bundles are typically hyper-sensitive to the slightest stimulation. Demyelinated nerves may become sites of spontaneous activity and develop connections with pain terminals from the dorsal horn of the spinal cord. This too may result in misintepre-tation of innocuous stimuli as painful (Inbal, 1987 and Woolf, 1992).

In fibromyalgia and other pain-related syndromes of Somatoneural Dysfunction, it appears that neuropathic pain occurs without nerve injury. Peripheral nerves generally appear normal on assessment of nerve conduc-tion velocity but manifest the same clinical and biochemical patterns as is seen with true nerve injury states. It is also possible that there is existing nerve injury in SND, but that it is below the threshold detectable my mod-ern medical testing. Because of the overall sensitization of the pain cascade in SND patients, this "subthreshold" injury is enough to cause significant symptomatology.

Sleep

Most researchers consider sleep a key component in the understanding and treatment of Somatoneural Dysfunction and its subtypes. There may be significant overlap between the types of abnormalities seen in SND and those of primary sleep disorders (such as narcolepsy and sleep apnea) and depression.

Normal sleep is characterized by two separate physiological states, called rapid eye movement (REM) and non-rapid eye movement (NREM). NREM sleep can be divided into stages 1 through 4 on the basis of brain wave patterns seen on an electroencephalogram (EEG). It is a state of drastically decreased physiologic activity. Roughly 25% of sleep is spent in the REM state, which generally occurs 90 minutes after the onset of sleep and is marked by a high level of brain and physiological activity that is similar to that seen during wakefulness (Kaplan and Sadock, 1998).

Normally, when people are awake, the EEG shows "alpha" waves, which are low voltage, random, and have a fast frequency. This does not hold true among members of The Grateful Dead, whose brains have developed a unique frequency called "Wavy Gravy". When people first fall asleep, the alpha wave pattern is replaced by a slower, more regular pattern, the theta wave. This quickly gives way to stage 2 sleep, typified by sleep spindles and K-complexes on the EEG. Nearly half of a night's sleep is spent in stage 2. High-voltage, high frequency delta waves then make their appearance in stages 3 and 4. This is commonly referred to as slow-wave sleep. The appearance of sleep as seen by the EEG is shown in Figure 3.

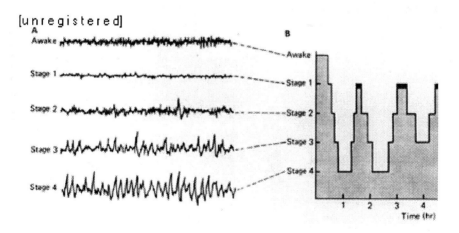

Normal NREM sleep is marked by a slow, regular pulse and rate of breathing, decreased blood pressure, closely regulated body temperature, and a relaxed muscle tone. Blood flow and metabolic activity is reduced in brain tissue, which can result in disorientation if awakened during the deeper stages of sleep. Cortisol and TSH (thyroid-stimulating hormone) secretion diminish with sleep onset and increase towards reawakening.

REM sleep is a time of heightened metabolic activity, similar to, and sometimes exceeding that of wakefulness. Bursts of intense brain activity occur during REM sleep, which generally appears several times during a nights sleep intermixed with slow-wave sleep. This activity is manifested clinically as rapid eye movements in all directions and twitching of facial muscles and other small muscle groups. The pupils alternately dilate and constrict and there are dramatic variations in breathing, heart rate, and blood pressure. People dream mainly during REM sleep and penile erections occur. The muscles are limp and reflexes are diminished, but the brain seems to be working overtime, with increased metabolic activity and oxygen consumption. What on Earth is all this about?

Why Do We Sleep?

The brilliant physiologist Sir John Eccles observed as late as 1977 that "Sleep is a natural repeated unconsciousness that we do not even know the reason for" (Popper and Eccles, 1977). This is certainly true even as we enter the new millennium, and research into the physiologic function of sleep has barely scratched the surface. The standard clinical neurology textbook, *Principles of Neurology*, has a section on the function of sleep totaling 11 lines out of 1612 pages and concludes:

"The authors, on the basis of plausibility and logic, favor the simple notion that sleep restores strength and physical and mental energy" (Kandel and Schwartz, 2000).

One could assume that, since we spend roughly one third of our entire lives in the sleep state, we should know more about what goes on during that time. Yet, sleep research is really a product only of the last decade and has barely shed any light on the issue. At least one sleep physiologist has confided in me that he suspects that the mysteries of sleep hold the keys to virtually all human health, illness, and aging.

In animal studies, we have learned a few things that suggest the importance of sleep. Laboratory rats deprived of sleep die after about three weeks of sleep deprivation and after five weeks of being deprived of REM sleep. Sleep and its stages are also closely regulated; sleep deprivation is followed by sleep rebound and loss of certain stages of sleep result in compensatory increase in that stage when sleep does occur (Rechstaffen, 1998). Lastly, all species sleep (unless you count very low forms of life such as amoebas and telephone company telemarketers), despite the fact that it does not appear to serve a critical function in propagating the species. Somehow, we must be missing something that speaks to the importance of sleep.

NREM Sleep

The previously held belief that sleep is merely to rest and conserve energy has been essentially dismissed. People thought that NREM sleep in particular, where there is a reduction in energy expenditure, was just a time to recuperate from the day's activities. However, we have come to realize that the total metabolic activity in sleep is only reduced by ten percent or so, which is hardly worth wasting six or eight hours.

The main feature of brain function during NREM sleep seems to be that there is a different level of neuronal activity in different areas of the brain. High rates of periodic activity (burst-pause pattern) and increased function in the hypothalamus seems to indicate an attempt at fine-tuning the delicate system controlling hormone and neurotransmitter synthesis and regulation. The hypothalamus may be sending out these brief spikes of information in order to adjust the body's metabolic response.

Concurrent reductions in cortisol___and thyrotropin (which enhance metabolism) may be necessary to focus the brain's energy on adjustment instead of function.

The amygdala and basal forebrain are involved in

Table 2: Areas of the Brain with Increased Activity During NREM Sleep
Hypothalamus: hormone control
Amygdala: mood and emotion
Basal Forebrain: emotion
Nucleus Solitarius: sympathetic nervous system

emotion, and some theorize that NREM sleep functions as"natural psychotherapy" to keep us centered and sane. The nucleus solitarius plays a major role in regulating sympathetic control of the adrenal gland and the cardiovascular system. Increased metabolic hormones (particularly growth hormone) may play a role in this regulatory process as well. The parasympathetic nervous system probably acts to tone down the body's activity in order to direct energy towards these regulatory functions.

Table 3: Features of NREM Sleep

Brain Activity
   Reduced cerebral metabolism during slow wave sleep
   Variation in cerebral blood flow and neuronal activity
   Burst-pause firing pattern in several brain areas
   Sleep-active neurons in hypothalamus, amygdala,
         forebrain, and nucleus of the solitary tract
   Neuron hyperpolarization

Endocrine Features
   Increased glucose, growth hormone, insulin, aldosterone
   Increased prolactin and testosterone
   Reduced cortisol and thyrotropin

Systemic features
   Parasympathetic dominance
   Decreased brain and body temperature

REM Sleep

Humans generally spend about two hours in REM sleep at regular 90-minute intervals interspersed throughout the night. However, the function of REM sleep may be even more perplexing. It appears to be physiologically a state of arousal similar to waking. Why, then, don't we just wake up?

Table 4: Features of REM Sleep

Body Features
> Rapid eye movements
> Irregular heart rate, respiration, and blood pressure
> Penile erections
> Decreased temperature regulation
> Alternating vasodilatation and vasoconstriction
> Increased whole body metabolic rate

Brain Features
> Abundant dreaming
> Increased cerebral metabolism and blood flow
> Increased brain temperature and intracranial pressure
> Increased neuronal activity in the pons, visual cortex, pyramidal tract, reticular formation,
> > Reticular formation, and lateral tegmentum
> Decreased neuronal activity in the raphe nucleus and locus coerulus
> Hippocampal hyperactivity

First of all, dreams occur during REM sleep. Sigmund Freud was one of the first to analyze dreams as having important impact on our waking lives. He theorized that we dream to help us interpret and deal with the trials and tribulations of our waking life. Somehow, he thought, our subconscious speaks to us in suggestions or warnings through dreams.

Obviously, the increases in brain metabolic activity and blood flow indicate that something important is going on. Psychiatrists and sleep theorists have used the relationship between brain activity and the most obvious manifestation of this activity, the dream, to reflect on its importance. Some say that dreams are critical to emotional adaptation and stability.

All of the areas that have increased activity in the REM state are involved in dreaming. The similarities between the sleeping and waking states in this regard can help explain why some dreams seem so real. Serotonin and norepinephrine are intimately involved in dream production, so it is possible that the other areas of the brain with high activity of these neurotransmitters (raphe nucleus and locus coerulus) may be turned down to prevent interference. Lastly, the hyperactivity in the hippocampus during REM sleep is probably an indication of memory consolidation and retention.

Overall, sleep seems to be important in emotion and memory and serves as a bridge to the subconscious. This is part of what makes us who we are during the day! It is easy to envision that drastic abnormalities in sleep and sleep stages can have a significant impact on our lives during the day. In Somatoneural Dysfunction, this important regulatory mechanism is usually disrupted and unable to help correct other metabolic and emotional disturbances.

The Immune System

In naming Somatoneural Dysfunction, I tried to impart the notion of a defect of the way somatic sensations (pain, fatigue, etc.) are processed and interpreted by the central nervous system. In doing so, I left out direct reference to a number of other systems involved in the disorder. I suppose to correctly label this disorder, I should call it "Somatopsychoimmunoendogastrorheumagastroneural Dysfunction", but then no one would buy this book. So I shortened it.

That is not to say, however, that the other involved systems are any less important, especially the immune system. For centuries, the immune system was thought to be distinctly separate from the other systems of the body. Rene Descartes, the famous 17th century French scientist, erroneously concluded that the mind and the body were completely separate entities. He reached this conclusion more in part, I believe, due to threats from the Church that jeapordized the connection of his brain to his neck, rather than rigorous scientific theory. This error was perpetuated, unfortunately, until about the 1970s and was not firmly contradicted until a landmark study in 1981.

The immune system is essentially composed of two lines of defense for protection of the body from dangerous cells, which may come from the outside (viruses, bacteria, allergens, etc.) or from the inside (cancer cells). The cells of the immune system that protect us from these dangers originate in the bone marrow and are divided into two types: T-cells and B-cells. T-cells (the T stands for "thymus", which is an organ prominent mainly in embryonic development where the cells matured) function in cellular immunity. This system has many different cell types that act directly to destroy harmful invaders.

Neutrophils (involved predominantly in fighting off bacterial infections) go directly to the site of attack and destroy infecting cells by phagocytosis or toxin release. Phagocytosis is the process of eating the harmful cells, digesting them, and spitting them out. No, really! Toxin release may damage or kill infecting cells, but can also be quite annoying to the patient as well. This is essentially what is responsible for the runny nose associated with a cold and the redness that can occur at the site of an infected cut.

Lymphocytes are important in fighting off infections by viruses, as well as other infections and cancers. It is a special type of T-cell (the CD4 or helper T-cell) that is destroyed by the HIV virus that causes AIDS. This renders AIDS patients extremely susceptible to viral, parasitic, and fungal infections as well as certain types of cancers. These cells are also defective in some types of hematologic malignancies, such as leukemia. Lympho-cytes can also release toxins and phagocytize invading cells, but primarily serve to control and regulate other aspects of the immune defense system.

Eosinophils are the primary armament versus allergic attacks. An allergy is designed to evoke a defensive response when the body encounters something it sees as foreign or harmful. Normally, the allergy defense system is triggered by an irritant (like pollen, ragweed, or Newt Gingrich). It may also be incited by a cancer or an infection. The problem is that many other things may appear to the allergy system as harmful when they really aren't. Thus someone may be allergic to innocuous substances like peanuts or seafood, helpful things like penicillin or a kidney transplant, or even parts of their own body (autoimmunity).

Other cells, such as the menacingly named natural killer (NK) cells act nonspecifically in attacking any type of threat to the body. These cells originate mainly in the bone marrow and circulate through the vascular and lymphatic systems searching out enemies to attack. The lymphatic system is a series of connections that usually course alongside or connect with blood vessels. The lymph nodes and other organs of the lymphatic system (tonsils, appendix, spleen) serve as a filtering system for the by-products of the "battles" of the immune system.

The other arm of the immune system is called the humoral immune system and is comprised mainly of antibodies. Antibodies, sometimes called immunoglobulins by people wearing white coats, are formed by B-cells (named because they originally matured in the bone marrow) and plasma cells in response to infection or allergy. They serve a variety of functions, such as attracting other cells to the site of attack, remembering harmful invaders in order to enhance the immune attack if they are seen again, and helping to destroy attacking cells directly. Antibodies may coat an invading cell in order to make it easier for T-cells to destroy, or even punch holes in the cell walls of intruding organisms to render them harmless.

Antibodies are said to be specific. In essence, the body develops antibodies against every harmful thing a person is exposed to (although not, unfortunately to things like Booger Bailey, the big kid that stole my lunch money in third grade). Antibodies remember harmful stimuli and act more aggressively if exposed again. Sometimes this is beneficial, resulting in immunity to chicken pox after your initial infection. Sometimes it is not, as when an anaphylactic reaction occurs the second time you're stung by a bee if you are allergic. Anaphylaxis is the immune system gone haywire in a desperate attempt to rid one of an offending toxin.

Defects

Defects in the immune system, caused either by infections like HIV, cancers like leukemia, chronic diseases such as diabetes, or genetic defects, make a person very susceptible to infections. I had a patient the other day call me hysterically worried because she had visited her boyfriend's grandfather in the hospital. Apparently, this unfortunate gentleman (who was in his nineties and suffered from lung cancer, diabetes, and kidney failure) died of viral pneumonia and my patient was afraid she was going to be very sick as a result. She, of course, was unlikely to become extremely ill as a result of exposure to this virus. The same virus that killed her boyfriend's grandfather would give her a cold at worst. A young, healthy person with a normally functioning immune system would have no trouble in fending off a virus that was deadly to someone with a malfunctioning immune system.

The immune system may also become defective and attack a person's own cells. There are many different types of autoimmune diseases where this occurs. In systemic lupus erythematosus (Lupus or SLE), many different autoantibodies are formed and can attack a variety of cells in the skin, kidneys, or connective tissue. Rheumatoid arthritis probably occurs as a result of T-supressor cell malfunction. These cells are supposed to turn off the immune response when it is no longer needed, but become defective in RA and lead to destruction of the connective tissue in joints by the patient's own immune cells. Multiple sclerosis may be an autoimmune disorder as well, characterized by destruction of white matter nerve cells in the brain by the immune system.

The reason why these autoimmune defects occur is still controversial and under investigation. The most likely explanation is that the immune system is tricked into thinking the body's own cells are harmful by previous exposure to viruses or allergens. For example, if you are exposed to virus X, your immune system may make antibodies to a molecule on the coating of the viral cell in order to attack and defend against it. This molecule may look very similar to a molecule on cells within the islets of Langerhans in your pancreas. Your immune system may then destroy these islet cells, thinking they are again under attack by virus X. This can result in type I diabetes.

The immune system works closely with the other organ systems of the body to maintain health and well-being. As we shall see, abnormalities and strains on immune system function play an important role in the development of Somatoneural Dysfunction.

The Connection Between the Brain and Illness

The notion that psychological input from the brain has an important impact on the development and recovery from disease and injury is not a new one. Lucius Seneca, a Stoic writing about two thousand years ago, stated "it is part of the cure to wish to be cured". Many of our grandmothers knew this connection and said, "you'll worry yourself sick!" The power of the mind is indeed extraordinary, as Harvard physiologist Walter Cannon found in the 1940s investigating claims of voodoo in rural Louisiana. He concluded people could die from "the fatal power of the imagination working through unmitigated terror". The mind's ability to control bodily functions is mediated mainly through noradrenergic connections within the autonomic nervous system, but a whole host of neurotransmitters, hormones, and peptides are involved.

The scientific community did not have firmevidence of the link between the central nervous system and the immune system until 1981, when researchers found definitive evidence that there were receptors for neurotransmitters released from the nervous system present on lymph-ocytes. In the ensuing two decades, the central nervous system control of immune system components has been firmly established and mapped (Ader, 1991).

Close your eyes and imagine you are holding a lemon. You can feel its bumpy surface and know its bright yellow in color. Imagine how it feels as you peel back the skin to reveal the pulpy fruit beneath. Now imagine yourself taking a bite and taste the bitter taste on your tongue.

Did you find yourself salivating at the thought of the lemon? Congratulations, you have first hand evidence of the brain's control over a complex bodily function.

Still, researchers could not accept the fact that psychological factors also play an important role in immune system function. Until that is, a group of researchers at the University of Rochester put their heads together to tackle the issue. Robert Ader (a psychiatrist), David Felten (a neurobiologist), and Nicholas Cohen (an immunologist) were able to establish that a "psychosomatic" process could even occur in laboratory animals to affect the course of a deadly autoimmune disease. Imagine how you would go about researching the question of whether psychologic factors could influence the immune systems of laboratory rodents. Pretty difficult, I presume? Well, only a little luck and the combined brilliance of such an interdisciplinary team could have solved this question.

In 1974, Dr. Ader was investigating the conditioned response of laboratory animals. Many decades before, Pavlov had shown that he could couple the sound of a bell with the idea of food and induce salivation in dogs (much like the little lemon exercise above, but with a bell). Ader wanted to find out how long this conditioning would last. He combined sweet tasting saccharine with the chemotherapy drug cyclophosphamide, a chemical that induces severe nausea in rats (as well as humans). He found that the animals began to die of infections and tumors if they continued to be given saccharine without the cyclophosphamide. The small dose of cyclophosphamide used in the conditioning response if given alone had no such effect (Ader, 1991).

With Felten's discovery of nerve contact with immune cells and tissue and Cohen's expertise in immune system function, the trio formulated one of the most interesting studies of the last century in the early 1980s in Rochester.

Using a certain strain of mice that were genetically afflicted with a deadly autoimmune disease (similar in nature to Lupus in humans), the group documented conditioned immunosuppression. The immune system of these mice normally attacks their own cells, particularly in the kidney, and caused kidney failure and death, usually within 24 months. In this case, the mouse's enemy was its own immune system and the immunosuppressant cyclophosphaminde actually increases the mouse's health and survival.

The study divided the mice into four groups. There were two control groups, one that received saccharine alone and another that received treatment with cyclophosphamide for 12 months. The first group lived an average of 24 months, and developed renal injury by 18 months. The second group's lives were extended by the cyclophosphamide to an average of 36 months, delaying the onset of renal injury by about a year. The two study groups were each given six months of cyclophosphamide. The first study group received no conditioning stimulus

> Group 1: Saccharine for 12 months
>   Lives 24 months
>
> Group 2: Cyclophosphamide for 12 months
>   Lives 36 months
>
> Group 3: Saccharine for 6 months + cyclophosphamide for 6 months
>   Lives 30 months
>
> Group 4: Saccharine + cyclo-phosphamide for 6 months, then saccharine for 6 months

and lived an average of 30 months, six months longer than the mice with-out any treatment, but not as long as those receiving a full course of ther-apy, as one would expect. The interesting finding came in the other group, which was conditioned to actually "think" it had received a full 12 months of treatment.

The researchers went back to Ader's original model of conditioning and coupled the taste of saccharine with the injection of cyclophosphamide. After six months, investigators stopped the medication, but continued the saccharine. How long did these mice live? Almost 36 months, just about as long as the mice that had received twice as much medication. What on earth does that mean?

Well, to start, it means that somehow the mice thought that the sac-charine was making them better and continued to get better when given saccharine alone. This connection was even able to overcome the aversive stimuli of a painful injection and the nausea that accompanied the cyclo-phosphamide. The mouse's brain thought the saccharine was making it better, so it got better. This resulted from direct connections from the brain to the immune system and showed that a message from the brain could override immune system function.

This study also serves to explain the placebo effect where patients sometimes may gain some benefit in symptoms or disease states from treatments with no biological activity, such as sugar pills. Some of the most striking evidence of the effectiveness of the placebo came from wartime anecdotes of injured soldiers. On several occasions, particularly during World War II, medics treating badly injured soldiers would run out of morphine pain reliever and would give injections or saline instead. Amazingly, the medics would often return to find their wounded patients sleeping comfortably without benefit from any real pain medicine.

The placebo response stemming from positive belief mechanisms is very powerful and should not be viewed lightly. It is probably responsible for benefits seen from therapies such as homeopathic remedies that have no real biological activity.

The Endocrine System

The endocrine system is defined by Merriam-Webster's Dictionary as, "the glands and parts of glands that produce endocrine secretions, help to integrate and control bodily metabolic activity, and include especially the pituitary, thyroid, parathyroids, adrenals, islets of Langerhans, ovaries, and testes. The term "endocrine" simply refers to a substance (usually a hormone) that is released by a gland and exerts an effect on a distant site. It has often been said that if doctors have no idea what is wrong with a patient, the condition usually involves the endocrine system. Hence it comes as no surprise that the endocrine system is also involved in Somatoneural Dysfunction. This involvement occurs mainly in the hypo-thalamic-pituitary-adrenal system, which impacts on virtually every other organ system in the body.

The top of the system is the hypothalamus, which can be viewed as the control center for homeostasis—the process of maintaining the normal function of all the body's systems. It receives direct input from the cerebral cortex as well as information from the target organs under its control. This latter "feedback loop" allows the hypothalamus to know what is going on downstream and correct and regulate any disturbances in the status quo.

The anterior pituitary, under instruction from the hypothalamus via releasing hormones, in turn controls the functioning of the thyroid, adrenal glands, and ovaries or testes. It also releases prolactin (responsible for breast development for nursing after pregnancy), growth hormone (which guides cell growth and development), lipotropin (a poorly understood hormone that may play a role in metabolism and energy storage), and endorphins (involved in pain perception and control). The hormones and their target organs are listed in table 5.

Table 5: Hormones and their Effects

Pituitary Hormone	Target Organ
Growth hormone	Liver, muscle, bone
Prolactin	Breast
Thyroid-stimulating hormone (TSH)	Thyroid
Follicle-stimulating hormone (FSH)	Ovaries/testes
Luteinizing hormone (LH)	Ovaries/testes
Adrenocorticotropin hormone (ACTH)	Adrenal glands
Lipotropin	Fat cells
Endorphin	Nerve cells

Follicle-stimulating hormone and luteinizing hormone play important roles in male and female sexual development and function. In males, they act on the testes to release testosterone from the Leydig cells and spermatozoa from the seminiferous tubules. In females, FSH and LH regulate the ovarian cycle and allow the formation and release of estrogen and progesterone.

In addition to the obvious effects of maintaining sexual reproduction, development, and activity, testosterone and estrogen serve a number of other functions as well. Testosterone is involved in the maintenance of muscle and bone mass, energy, skin, hair texture and distribution, and prostate health. In women, estrogen is also involved in maintaining bone density (deficiency of estrogen predisposes to osteoporosis), cardiovascular health, menstrual function, and skin and connective tissue preservation.

The Thyroid

The thyroid gland sits in the middle of your neck, wrapped snugly around your trachea. Its function, in a nutshell, is the body's metabolism. Receptors for thyroid hormone are found in virtually all tissues in the body, and its effects at the cellular level are quite complex. Hyperfunction of the thyroid is not usually seen in conjunction with Somatoneural Dysfunction, but there may be concurrent hypothyroidism or altered functioning of the thyroid hormone system. A look at the possible symptoms of hypothyroidism can demonstrate the complexity and broad spectrum of impact of thyroid function.

Table 6: Hypothyroidism: The Great Mimicker (Robins, 2000)

Neuropsychiatric	Dementia, dysarthria, deafness, ataxia, peripheral neuropathy, carpal tunnel syndrome, neuroses, psychoses
Cardiopulmonary	Hypertension, heart failure, enlarged heart, fluid buildup in the heart or lungs, respiratory depression
Gastrointestinal	Constipation, ascites, ileus
Genitourinary	Impotence, menstrual irregularity, premenstrual syndrome
Musculoskeletal	Joint pain, muscle aches or cramps
Hematologic	Anemia
Endocrine	Growth retardation, fluid imbalance
Metabolic	Liver injury, increased cholesterol, increased calcium or uric acid
General	Fatigue, weight gain

What is actually most common in SND is "subclinical hypothyroidism". This is a state where there is an elevated TSH, but normal levels of circulating thyroid hormones. These so-called normal levels are just not normal for the individual patient with SND who is sensitive to the metabolic activities of these hormones. The range of normal for TSH can vary from 0.5 to 5, a full ten-fold difference. Simply put, for many patients, especially those with SND, what is normal for most, may not be normal for you. The brain is trying to tell us that by releasing more TSH.

The Adrenal Glands

One adrenal gland sits atop each kidney, relatively small and unobtrusive. However, it plays an extremely important role in maintaining the body's homeostatic mechanisms as well. It consists of two parts: the medulla and the cortex. The adrenal medulla is really a part of the autonomic nervous system, receiving input via nerve endings containing predominantly norepinephrine and releasing epinephrine in response. Epinephrine is the main signaler in the "fight or flight" response and has a wide variety of biological effects designed to get you out of danger.

During evolution, this epinephrine emergency response system developed in order to increase blood pressure, heart rate, and respiratory rate in order to deliver more blood and oxygen to muscles so that you could run faster or fight better. In doing so, it shunts blood and oxygen away from tissues and organs that aren't as important in fighting or flighting: mainly the skin and gastrointestinal tract. It also sends reminders to the brain that "maybe you should get the heck out of here" by causing feelings of anxiety or impending doom. Overstimulation of this system can lead to chest pain, headache, and palpitations, hallmark signs of a panic attack.

The adrenal cortex secretes two important substances in response to commands from the brain and input from the vascular system in a feedback loop: aldosterone and cortisol. Aldosterone is responsible for maintaining the body's delicate balance of volume status and electrolytes, particularly sodium and potassium. It works closely with parts of the kidney to perform this function and is also involved in blood pressure control.

Cortisol is secreted mainly in response to ACTH (adrenocorticotropin hormone) from the pituitary and is also influenced by daily rhythms and stress (keep that in mind!). Cortisol has a critical permissive role in protein breakdown, nitrogen excretion, fat deposition, and appetite. It increases glucose production in the liver by mobilizing amino acids stored in bone, muscle, connective tissue, and other organs and serves to inhibit use of glucose in target organs. Furthermore, it has important roles in optimizing cardiovascular function, assisting in the kidney's ability to control fluids and volume, and enhancing central nervous system activity.

Cortisol plays a dramatic role in the immune system and the inflammatory response. It inhibits inflammation and decreases swelling. This is desirable to lessen the effects of tissue injury, but can serve to worsen infection by decreasing the body's natural defenses. It can actually shut down the immune response by impairing the ability of white blood cells to migrate to the site of inflammation or infection and preventing them from destroying bacteria. This is part of the body's natural "shut-down" mechanism designed to turn off the immune and inflammatory response when it is no longer needed. Many drugs have been developed that are similar in effect to the body's own cortisol, such as dexamethasone, prednisone, cortisone, and hydrocortisone. They have similar beneficial and detrimental effects on patients as natural cortisol.

Deficiency or failure of the adrenal cortex can result in weakness, fatigue, poor appetite, low blood pressure, menstrual irregularity, gastrointestinal distress, muscle cramps, and electrolyte disturbances among many other symptoms. If this sounds familiar, it should. Many believe this powerful gland is also involved in the pathogenesis of Somatoneural Dysfunction.

Stress

Now that we, and the rest of the scientific community, agree that the brain is able to exert direct control on the immune system, we should explore how this can be detrimental as well as potentially beneficial. Thus we have actually come back to grandmother's idea that worrying too much could lead to increased susceptibility to illness. In fact, she was right.

We have known for decades that psychological stress exerts a number of effects. Studies done on cardiovascular disease in the seventies revealed that highly stressed patients, so-called "type A", had an increased risk for heart attacks. Stress in can cause sugar levels to rise in diabetics, can increase your chance of getting an ulcer, and undoubtedly contributes to increased severity in depression and anxiety disorders.

As I mentioned a little while ago, stress play as regulatory role in cortisol release from the adrenal cortex. It is through the activity of cortisol that stress exerts most of its activities on the body. Release of epinephrine from the autonomic nervous system is another mechanism influenced by stress. This can lead to a state of neurologic hyperresponsiveness and cause the central nervous system to react more forcefully to disturbances in its delicate regulatory processes. In addition to those effects listed above, stress impacts on health and illness through its influence on the immune system.

Researchers at The Ohio State University College of Medicine have been studying two groups of highly stressed individuals. To look at the effects of acute stress, they evaluated medical students around the time of final exams, and to address the issue of chronic stress, caregivers of Alzheimer's Disease patients were studied. They looked at both clinical findings and biologic and chemical changes within the body.

The medical students generally reported increased symptoms of anxiety, depression, and illness such as cold or flu symptoms around the time of exams. When their immune systems were studied, researchers found decreased ability of immune cells to fight off infection, decreased reaction of immune cells to viruses, lessened antibody response, and increased reactivation of dormant viruses such as herpes or Epstein-Barr virus. This is why you cold sores seem to recur around the time your mother-in-law visits...

Caregivers showed similar changes in immune function. In addition, they also showed an increased level of ACTH, implicating an enhanced cortisol secretion as a result of chronic stress. When investigators looked at wound healing in these same caregivers, they discovered that it took almost 25% longer for wounds to heal that in their "nonstressed" counterparts (Glaser, 1998).

Stress reduction has been, despite convincing studies like these, a largely overlooked area of treatment and health maintenance.

Other Symptoms of Somatoneural Dysfunction and Why They Occur

There are a whole bunch of symptom complexes that appear over and over in SND patients and reflect certain abnormalities in biological function. This is another reason why narrow definitions like the ACR guidelines for fibromyalgia and the CDC criteria for chronic fatigue syndrome do not adequately express the variety of symptoms that may occur.

Dr. Starlanyl's book lists no fewer than 94 individual symptoms that may occur in patients with fibromyalgia/myofascial pain syndrome and even goes as far as to correctly call it a "sensitivity-amplification syndrome" and "Irritable Everything Syndrome". Inexplicably, she maintains the belief that the abnormalities lie in the myofascia and not in the central nervous system. The myofascia just sits there minding its own business while the painful information it transmits are wrongly interpreted by the CNS. Similarly, other sensory information (position, pressure, temperature, etc) also causes overreactivity in the central nervous system. This is how such a wide variety of symptoms can occur in an individual patient.

Just to summarize, I will divide the symptoms in five main categories:

1) Abnormalities in pain processing
2) Sleep disturbances
3) Abnormalities in the endocrine systems
4) Immune system dysfunction
5) Coexisting stress-related disorders

We have already seen how abnormalities in pain processing can lead to myofascial tender points, painful muscle spasms, headaches, generalized achiness, low back pain, and neuropathic pains. Patients may also experience temporo-mandibular joint dysfunction, Eustachian tube dysfunction and chronic ear pain, chronic pelvic pain and dyspareunia (pain during intercourse). Similar problems with interpreting sensory input may lead to dizziness or balance difficulties, although this should always prompt a search for other causes.

Sleep disturbances such as restless leg syndrome, nocturnal leg cramps, and sleep apnea may occur. Of course, dysfunctional sleep patterns contribute to overall worsening of fatigue and most other symptoms of SND by failing to replenish needed homeostatic resources.

Endocrine problems obviously contribute to fatigue, but may also cause symptoms such as carbohydrate-craving due to a sensitivity to low levels of glucose, difficulty maintaining normal weight, and fluctuation in or difficulty maintaining normal blood pressure.

Immune system dysfunction can lead not only to susceptibility to infections (particularly viral and yeast infections), but to sensitivity in other areas as well. Patients with SND may be overly sensitive to medications and allergens. They may also have dry or itchy skin, a chronic runny or stuffy nose, or chronic cough due to sensitivity to inflammatory mediators.

Finally, stress-related disorders can lead to difficulty with concentration or memory (so-called "fibrofog"), depression, anxiety, panic attacks. In fact, since we all agree this is a "sensitivity-amplification syndrome" any other disease or medical problem that a patient has will be made worse by the SND. This is an important point to remember when reflecting on treatment approaches, since not only does the specific medical problem need to be treated, but the SND as well.

Other Symptoms

Not a lot of attention has been focused on other symptoms of Somatoneural Dysfunction. None of them find their way into the diagnostic criteria for fibromyalgia, chronic fatigue syndrome, or any other related disorder. Despite this, if you get a bunch of people with these disorders together, you will find certain common symptom patterns.

Fibrofog

Fibrofog refers to a common complaint of fibromyalgia patients that they are confused, or have problems writing or reading by misplacing words, or feel a sense of depersonalization. Of course, it is not limited to fibromyalgia, but may be seen in chronic fatigue syndrome or any other type of Somatoneural Dysfunction. It is a feeling difficult for patient and physician to describe. Dr. Devin Starlanyl tries in vain in her book, quoting several patients (Starlanyl, 1996):

"Why isn't whatever I'm looking for where I thought I put it?"

"With fibrofog you're in a game where the rules keep changing and nobody tells you what they are."

"Sometimes I feel like my body is just a shell, and I'm only dust inside"

And so on.

Abnormalities associated with fibrofog can be divided into three main categories: disorder of memory, disorder of consciousness, and disorder of concentration. True memory disorders are relatively rare in Somatoneural

Dysfunction and their presence should always trigger a search for other causes. True loss of long term memory leads to forgetting your way home or the names of your children and such things.

Disorders of consciousness such as a feeling of depersonalization or detachment from ones' life or surroundings is a much better sign of a coexisting depressive or anxiety disorder than of SND. It can be brought on or worsened by many medications commonly used to treat these conditions such as pain relievers, antidepressants, or anti-anxiety medications.

What is usually seen in SND is a difficulty in concentrating and a defect in short term memory. The typical SND patient is distracted by stressful life events and medical illness, which is worsened by lack of sleep and medication use. Patients have trouble remembering what they went into the kitchen to get. They can't remember phone numbers or things on their grocery list and have trouble organizing things at work. The problem becomes frustrating and leads to more anxiety, which of course, worsens the initial problem. Fibrofog can sometimes be the most disabling aspect of SND.

Vertigo

Many patients with Somatoneural Dysfunction, suffer from problems with balance or dizziness. Balance is a complicated neurologic process involving communication between the brain and the vestibular apparatus (balance center) in the inner ear. Other sensory processes such as vision, vibration sense, and touch, as well as the cardiovascular system, contribute as well.

The semicircular canals in the ear are fluid filled structures that provide positional information to the brain via nerve transmitters. If you picture a carpenter's level with a little air bubble that moves when you change its angle, you won't be too far off. When the head is moved around, so does the fluid in three interlocked semicircular canals. How the fluid moves in three dimensions is picked up by nerve fibers and sent to the brain for interpretation.

This is quite a delicate and complicated little system. If the sensors, receptors, and transmitters don't talk properly, balance problems occur. In normal circumstances, the system adapts to minor abnormalities quite well. In SND, however, normal compensatory mechanisms are strained, making the problem difficult to correct and symptoms appear at relatively mild abnormalities.

Vasomotor Rhinitis

Patients with various types of Somatoneural Dysfunction commonly complain of chronic nasal or sinus conditions. They are always stuffy or runny or both. Quite often they are diagnosed with sinus infections and are treated with course after course of antibiotic, which only serves to make things worse by eliminating normal bacterial flora and contributing to antibiotic resistance.

So How Does This All Add Up to Somatoneural Dysfunction?

I believe that these pervasive abnormalities develop as a result of cumulative stresses to these delicately balanced systems in susceptible individuals. There is probably a genetic predisposition, since SND tends to run in families. Since nitric oxide seems to be involved in many or all of the above-mentioned abnormalities, it's quite possible that defects on the chromosome responsible for coding for nitric oxide metabolism is the culprit.

These individuals go through life encountering various traumatic events, both physical and psychological. These may be medical illnesses, viral or bacterial infections, physical trauma, or mental insult. The system compensates for each trauma as best it can until it becomes overwhelmed at a specific threshold. Then, the symptoms of Somatoneural Dysfunction begin to occur.

Each individual manifests symptom complexes differently in SND, the same as in every other disease. Cases may be more or less severe and present in a wide variety of ways depending on each individual's genetic, biological, and psychological makeup. We must also keep this in mind as we discuss treatments in the future.

Chapter 3:
Clinical Aspects of Somatoneural Dysfunction

Not Everything is Somatoneural Dysfunction

H.M. was a 70 year-old female who was referred to my office with the diagnosis of fibromyalgia. She had been diagnosed by her rheumatologist, who had been practicing the specialty for over 20 years and was very well- respected in the community. Mrs. M's primary care physician had cared for her for the previous six years. She had always had a bit of osteoarthritis, but when she began to develop progressively worsening pains in her joints over the last three years, her doctor sent her to an orthopedic specialist at the local community hospital as well as to a rheumatology consultant.

The orthopedist took a number of x-rays of her hips and knees, where the pain seemed to be worse, and diagnosed osteopenia. A subsequent densitometry scan confirmed severe osteoporosis and she was treated with anti-inflammatories, calcium, and a medicine to decrease the long-term effects of her thinning bones. When she developed acute back pain two years later, another orthopedic specialist, this time at a prestigious university hospital, diagnosed her with a vertebral compression fracture and started her on Percocet™, a strong narcotic pain reliever.

The patient and her family grew increasingly distressed because she had progressed to the point of constant pain, with frequent flares that were excruciating. Her doctors noted that she had an elevated level of calcium in her blood and attributed it to her calcium supplementation. Her poor protein levels and increased immunoglobulins were written off as due to poor nutrition and vitamin deficiency.

Mrs. M. became depressed and was referred to a psychiatrist, who started her on antidepressant therapy. Her rheumatologist sent her for physical therapy, but she was unable to participate due to her pain, despite taking morphine and Valium™. She tried to tell her doctor this, but he said she was "noncompliant" and not trying hard enough. She was tired all the time, but couldn't sleep due to the terrible pain. She was treated with steroids, underwent epidural injections and nerve blocks, and in desperation, saw a hypnotist and an herbalist. Her rheumatologist finally diagnosed her with fibromyalgia and added a second antidepressant to her regimen.

Her niece happened to be an aide at the hospital where I work and knew that I saw a number of patients with fibromyalgia. She then sent her aunt to me for a second opinion regarding treatment for her condition. When she arrived in a wheelchair and looking twenty years older than her stated age, I began to wonder about her diagnosis. I had seen patients with fibromyalgia confined to wheelchairs due to muscle weakness and disuse from years of inactivity due to pain, but not many. When I searched for trigger points, I found them just like in the textbooks, in fact, I found them just about everywhere. As I examined further, I found they weren't really trigger points at all, but rather discovered that she experienced bitter pain wherever I touched.

Her husband handed me a set of three x-rays of her shoulder and a panel of blood tests from a few months back. That was all of her records they could get, he said, though I surmised that dozens of x-rays and hundreds of lab tests were done over the last few years. He looked at me imploringly and continued, "I hope you can help her". I told him I would look at the tests and be right back, hoping indeed that I would be able to offer some assistance.

I put the films up on our x-ray reader in our back room and was struck by the almost absolute blackness that showed up where the bones should be. One of my nurses commented on their strange appearance and I explained that the patient had extremely severe osteoporosis. But as I looked further, I had to believe it was the worst case of osteoporosis I had ever seen. The bones of her humerus and shoulder were completely gone, almost "punched out" in places and utterly destroyed.

With a sinking feeling I looked down at her blood tests and noted several abnormalities on the printout: very high calcium, anemia, renal insufficiency, and high immunoglobulin levels. I sighed to myself and returned to Mrs. M and her husband, who looked up hopefully and asked me if I knew how to help her fibromyalgia.

I never know what to say in these situations or how to explain this to a patient and her family, but somehow I always manage.

"Mrs. M. doesn't have fibromyalgia, sir", I began, "I think she has something called multiple myeloma. It's a malignancy in the blood that can cause the bones to erode and may be responsible for her pain."

When they asked, I gave hopeful replies about possible treatments and control of her symptoms, but I had never seen a case of myeloma this severe at presentation and could not hope for much from chemotherapy. We ended our visit with a prescription for a stronger pain reliever and instructions to call if more was needed. I ordered more confirmatory tests, but none were really necessary.

By the time I had received her records and found that some signs of myeloma had been present for months, and others for years, Mrs. M. was in the intensive care unit of our hospital. We tried aggressive chemotherapy and kept her as comfortable as possible, but soon our team of pulmonologists, cardiologists, and oncologists concluded that nothing could be done for Mrs. M. Her family, understandably shaken and distraught, agreed to take her off life support and provide her with hospice care. She lasted exactly one day.

How did this happen? Was I so smart that only I could make the diagnosis that the others missed? I don't think so. I've certainly never professed to be that smart and my wife reminds me all the time that I forget to take out the garbage or do the dishes if she doesn't prod me. The doctors that Mrs. M. saw were specialists, some of them practicing for more years than I've been alive, and others devoting years specifically to the study of bones and joints.

The problem here was that the diagnosis of fibromyalgia was made without making sure everything else was definitively ruled out. Her symptoms certainly fit fibromyalgia, but the laboratory abnormalities and x-ray findings did not. Problems continued to persist because her doctors blamed every new finding on fibromyalgia, a common and inexcusable error. I ask one of my students one day if a patient with Somatoneural Dysfunction came into the emergency room with an axe sticking out of the back of their head if he would say, "must be that darn fibromyalgia acting up again…"

I stress to the residents and students that I teach that Somatoneural Dysfunction is a diagnosis of exclusion. This means that physicians must make every attempt to rule out other illnesses that may have similar symptoms. It is never possible to "rule in" SND, despite efforts by some groups to come up with unifying diagnostic criteria.

Some clinicians and myself have come up with a standard set of tests to do when the diagnosis of SND is suspected. Since there is no test to confirm or refute the diagnosis of SND directly, we strive to eliminate other disorders as diagnostic possibilities. A list of disorders with similar features is found in tables 7A-C, while a set of suggested tests for patients with suspected Somatoneural Dysfunction can be seen in table 8. Despite the fact that chronic fatigue accounts for over seven million office visits to physicians each year, the medical profession is still not very adept at diagnosing and treating these related conditions. I recommend a standard approach to the evaluation and management of Somatoneural Dysfunction that encompasses the general syndrome and all of its related disorders. I teach this section to medical students and residents, but believe that patients should also be educated on the appropriate workup for SND. In this manner, patients and their doctors will arrive at a mutual understanding of the presentation of the disorder and arrive at the correct diagnosis together, without missing other similar diseases.

Table 7A. Common Medical Causes of Chronic Fatigue

1. Infections
   - Intra-abdominal or intraspinal abscess
   - Chronic bacterial infections
     - Subacute bacterial endocarditis
     - Lyme Disease
     - Tuberculosis
   - Post-Infectious Syndromes
     - Brucellosis
     - Mononucleosis
   - Fungal
     - Histoplasmosis, blastomycosis, coccidioidomycosis
   - Parasitic
     - Toxoplasmosis, amebiasis
   - Human Immunodeficiency Virus (HIV) infection
2. Malignancies
   - Hematologic
     - Leukemias, multiple myeloma
   - Lymphoma/Hodgkin's Disease
   - Non-hematologic
     - Pancreatic, renal, gastric, lung, brain, and many others

3. Connective Tissue Disease
    - Rheumatoid arthritis
    - Polymyalgia Rheumatica
    - Sjogren's Syndrome, scleroderma
    - Subacute Lupus Erythematosus (SLE)
    - Granulomatous Diseases
      - Wegener's granulomatosis
      - Sarcoidosis
4. Endocrinopathies
    - Hypothyroidism
    - Diabetes mellitus
    - Cushing's syndrome (excess cortisol)
    - Adrenal insufficiency
5. Neuromuscular Diseases
    - Myasthenia gravis
6. Primary Seep Disorders
- Sleep apnea
- Narcolepsy and related syndromes
7. Drug/alcohol dependency or abuse
8. Neurologic Disorders
    - Multiple sclerosis, Parkinson's disease

Table 3B. Medications That Commonly Cause Fatigue

1. Pain Medication
    - Narcotics (morphine, hydrocodone, propoxyphene, etc)
    - Ultram
2. Tranquilizers
    - Benzodiazepines (diazepam, lorazepam, temazepam, alprazolam)
3. Cardiac Medications
    - ß-blockers (atenolol, metoprolol, etc)
    - Calcium-channel blockers (diltiazem, verapamil, amlodipine, etc)

- Centrally-acting agents (prazosin, reserpine, terazosin, clonidine)
4. Anti-depressants
   - Tricyclics (amitryptiline, nortryptiline, doxepin)
   - SSRIs (fluoxetine, paroxetine, sertraline)
   - Lithium
5. Anti-seizure Medications
   - Phenytoin, carbamazepine, valproic acid, phenobarbital, etc
6. Antihistamines
7. Muscle Relaxants

Table 3C. Psychiatric Disorders That May Cause Chronic Fatigue

1. Depression
   - Major depression
   - Dysthymia
2. Bipolar Disorder (Manic-Depression)
3. Anxiety Disorders
4. Panic Disorder
5. Somatoform Disorder

As you can see, this list covers quite a broad spectrum of pathology, though it is by no means exhaustive. Some of these disorders bear a brief explanation of the differences and similarities between them and Somatoneural Dysfunction.

Chronic infections have often been implicated in chronic fatigue and chronic fatigue syndromes in the past. The key to diagnosing chronic infection lies in the history and the ability to document a fever. One reason why the initial criteria established for chronic fatigue syndrome was changed was the inclusion of fever as one of the minor criteria. If a patient of mine has a fever greater than 100.6° F, I am concerned about infection, or in some cases malignancies, and set about on a directed search for the source. Lower grades of fever are common and may be part of the normal bodily variation throughout the day. As such, they are not a cause for concern.

Tuberculosis is a feared cause of chronic fatigue. If a patient has been exposed to tuberculosis at some point in their life, I will screen them with a PPD. Typically, patients with such exposure require yearly PPD placement to test for TB in any event. Toxoplasmosis is a parasitic infection often noted in cat owners or people who eat game meats. The discovery of lymph node enlargement causes suspicion for toxo, malignancy, or sarcoid and should always be evaluated. A biopsy should be performed if the lymph node enlargement is persistent.

Lyme Disease was thought to be involved in chronic fatigue syndrome for a while, but is really a well-defined clinical syndrome in its own right. Patients with frequent tick bites, particularly if the tick is discovered after a long period of time (more than a few hours), should be assessed for Lyme Disease. A characteristic "target lesion" rash called erythema chronicum migrans (red rash that comes and goes) is almost always present and should be a good diagnostic clue.

Malignancies are the most feared missed diagnosis of chronic fatigue. The best warning sign of malignancy is weight loss. Most patients with Somatoneural Dysfunction are inactive and thus have a hard time losing weight. Unintentional weight loss of more than ten pounds should be another signal for further investigation.

Rheumatologic diseases can often be difficult to diagnose, and should be screened for with laboratory testing. Painful joints that are warm, swollen, or red are often key diagnostic clues. Polymyalgia rheumatica in particular can be confused with SND because it shares many common characteristics. This is a low grade inflammatory disease of the muscles and joints and should be suspected in any elderly patient with an erythrocyte sedimentation rate greater than 50.

Low levels of thyroid hormone and high levels of glucose are associated with chronic fatigue, but often other clinical findings, such as thirst, constipation, frequent urination, or cold intolerance provide diagnostic clues.

Other hormone abnormalities, particularly affecting the hypothalamic-pituitary-adrenal axis can commonly present as fatigue as well.

Neurologic or neuromuscular disorders should be apparent on a thorough clinical exam, while alcohol and drug abuse should be screened for in a detailed history. The syndromes of narcolepsy and sleep apnea are becoming more and more frequently recognized as causes of chronic fatigue. Patients who fall asleep at the wheel or during conversations, or those who snore or awake with morning headaches should be assessed with a sleep study.

A detailed history of medication use should always be a part of the assessment. This includes over-the-counter remedies and herbal preparations, as their use is a common, and often overlooked, cause of chronic fatigue. Some of the medications used in the treatment of SND are listed above as possibly causing fatigue. They may, however, correct other biochemical disturbances that are at the root of the chronic fatigue of SND and may therefore actually improve fatigue when used appropriately.

Lastly, screening for psychiatric disorders should be done, but I disagree with the CDC guidelines that recommend it be done at the first visit. Since depression and other psychiatric disorders are also "diagnosed by exclusion" in patients who present with fatigue and other somatic complaints, this screening should be reserved until other diagnostic issues have been addressed.

Making The Diagnosis

It would be impossible for a general medical doctor or specialist to be expert in all of these areas of medicine. However, internal medicine and family practice physicians have a broad training and knowledge base and should know enough about each field to effectively assess and analyze the presence of most of these disorders in each patient. One of the most common ways for a patient to remain undiagnosed is to see a variety of different specialists without consulting a general practitioner who is better prepared to deal with the cross-specialty intricacies of Somatoneural Dysfunction.

The first step in the evaluation of a patient with suspected SND or simply one who presents with chronic fatigue is a review of previous medical records. A typical patient who is finally diagnosed with Somatoneural Dysfunction has seen, on average, six different physicians. The mean time of diagnosis for fibromylagia is 6.3 years and perhaps even longer for chronic fatigue syndrome. Obviously, the medical records of these patients may cover quite a lot of ground. Patients should forward a complete copy of their medical records for review at least a week prior to their appointment, and doctors should read them thoroughly before meeting the patient. Personally, I read these records the night before my appointments at the office or at home, and more often than not can reach a tentative diagnosis before even seeing the patient.

This saves time and limits fumbling through papers while trying to conduct a history and physical exam on a new patient. Unfortunately, I see many patients without benefit of prior records. Mr. L, a recent new patient with fibromyalgia, had seen 14 doctors in four states over a 17-year period before seeing me for his chronic fatigue. He hoped that I would be able to diagnose his ailment without benefit of the 650 pages of medical information that eventually accumulated at my office. Another problem is lack of effort on the part of previous physicians. Sometimes there is anger at losing a patient or a request for a second opinion, sometimes lack of promptness and inefficiency in busy offices, and often, lack of importance placed on forwarding the records of outgoing patients. On the rare occasion a patient leaves our practice, we send a complete copy of our charts the very same day. Patients need to provide a release form and request for record transfer in writing to every physician they have seen.

It saves time and effort if patients themselves have copies of their medical records. Patients with chronic medical problems, particularly one as complicated as Somatoneural Dysfunction, should update their medical file at six-month intervals or whenever they leave the practice of a given physician. I am unsure why this is not done more frequently. Perhaps some mystical stigma that says patients shouldn't look at their records remains. Once in a while I have left a patient's chart in the exam room and come back to "catch" them reading their chart. They always look guilty and sheepish, sometimes apologizing profusely. I immediately make a copy of the chart and give it to them with reassurance. It should be reiterated that the medical records are open to patients at any time and physicians cannot deny access to them at any time for any reason.

Without complete records, I am often forced to "start from scratch" and repeat laboratory, imaging, or diagnostic tests. This can be an aggravating and expensive process. No one wants to have another angiogram or colonoscopy just because the records were lost in transit. And, as a reminder, if your doctor dies or retires, get a copy of your records as soon as possible. I have experienced the "dead doctor dilemma" on quite a few occasions. This is like having your records eaten by your dog.

Once I have reviewed the records, I will meet with my new patient and take a thorough history of the problem, using the records as a guideline if at all possible. I then perform a physical exam directed by the history and previous findings. This examination varies from patient-to-patient, but always includes examination of the thyroid, lymphatic system, heart, lungs, abdomen, skin, musculoskeletal system, and a brief neurologic assessment. I also generally do trigger and tender point testing.

The Center for Disease Control recommends a mental status test for evaluation of chronic fatigue syndrome. I prefer the PRIME-MD tool, a 25-question device that can either be self-administered or given by a physician or nurse and takes an average of 8.4 minutes to perform. It is able to assess a patient's likelihood of having a significant mood, anxiety, eating, alcohol, or somatoform disorder and has an overall accuracy of 88% when compared with full psychiatric evaluation (Spitzer, 1994).

After this assessment I am able to fill in the blanks and schedule testing that may not have been checked previously in order to confirm or refute a potential diagnosis. I am usually then able to outline a potential treatment plan. This process should be standardized to practitioners across the country for evaluation of chronic fatigue and Somatoneural Dysfunction. If your doctor has omitted some parts of this, let him or her know!

Each patient with suspected SND should have an ALT (alanine aminotransferase) checked to screen for chronic liver disease, a creatinine level to test for kidney function, and a TSH (thyroid-stimulating hormone) to assess the function of the thyroid system. A CBC (complete blood count) should be checked to search for anemia and an abnormal white cell count that can sometimes accompany malignancies or chronic infections. An ESR (erythrocyte sedimentation rate) is usually assessed to screen for inflammatory processes, and an assessment of serum electrolytes (sodium, potassium, calcium, and phosphorous) and fasting glucose should be checked for excess or deficiency of sugar. The CDC also recommends a urinalysis, but I have not found this particularly useful.

I generally check an ANA (anti-nuclear antibody) and RA (rheumatoid arthritis) factor as part of a more complete screen for rheumatologic abnormalities. An SPEP (serum protein electrophoresis) can test for deficiency in proteins or immunoglobulins.

Other testing is dependent on the initial evaluation. An MRI (magnetic resonance imaging) scan of the brain or spinal cord may be useful in patients with focal neurologic findings. A sleep study or assessment of sleepiness called a Multiple Sleep Latency Test should be ordered if a primary sleep disturbance is suspected clinically. Suspicious lymph nodes or skin lesions often require antibiotic treatment or biopsy.

Any abnormalities on these initial tests should be followed up appropriately. For example, discovery of anemia should prompt assessment of iron stores, vitamin B12 and folate levels, and a search for occult blood loss.

Further invasive testing is usually not fruitful, adds drastically to the cost of the evaluation, and may result in unnecessary complications for the patient. Many tests are needless and may lead to other studies and treatments that are expensive, unnecessary, and even potentially dangerous.

This includes stool analysis, skin testing for food allergies, and cardiopulmonary exercise testing.

Table 8: Screening Tests to Assess Chronic Fatigue

CBC (complete blood count)
TSH (thyroid-stimulation hormone)
ALT (test of liver function)
ESR (erythrocyte sedimentation rate)
ANA (anti-nuclear antibodies)
RA-factor
Glucose (fasting if possible)
SPEP (serum protein immunoglobulins)
Creatinine (test of kidney function)
Electrolyte panel (sodium, potassium, chloride, and bicarbonate)
PRIME-MD

        Optional
Chest X-ray (in smokers)
Urinalysis
Magnesium, calcium, phosphate
Cortisol
Lyme titers
PPD (tes for exposure to tuberculosis)
Toxoplasma antibodies (IgG and IgM)
Sleep Studies
Uric Acid (elevated in gout)
Echocardiogram (if cardiac problems are suspected)
Plain X-rays
EMG/NCV (to assess for neuropathy)
HIV testing (in high risk individuals)
MRI of brain or spinal cord (if neurologic findings are noted on exam)

Chapter 4:

Related Disorders of Somatoneural Dysfunction

Chronic Fatigue Syndrome: Endocrine and Immunologic Defects in SND

In 1994, the Center for Disease Control, led by virologist Keiji Fukuda revised an earlier definition of chronic fatigue syndrome and set a new framework for future clinical research into pathogenesis, diagnosis, and treatment of the disease. They made several statements in addition to establishing criteria for diagnosis:

1) diagnosis of CFS can only be made after alternate medical and psychiatric causes of chronic fatiguing illness have been excluded
2) no pathognomonic (characteristic) signs or diagnostic tests for this condition have been established
3) no definitive treatment exists
4) most patients remain functionally impaired for several years (Fukuda, 1994)

This certainly doesn't lend much hope for this problem does it? They were essentially telling millions of people that they had an illness which couldn't be diagnosed, couldn't be treated, and that in all likelihood would result in suffering for several years. Thanks a lot! In the last five years or so, however, the picture has brightened a bit with a better understanding of chronic fatigue syndrome and its related conditions.

If we look at the original criteria for chronic fatigue syndrome proposed by the American College of Rheumatology in 1988, we can start to understand where some of the problems in diagnosis and treatment occurred. Holmes and coworkers (Holmes, 1988) stated that the fatigue in chronic fatigue syndrome had to meet a well-defined set of criteria, which was pretty hard to fulfill. The fatigue had to be of new onset without prior history of chronic fatigue and it had to result in greater than 50% reduction in the level of activity of the patient for greater than six months. It could not resolve with bed rest and all other medical and psychiatric illnesses had to be excluded.

Activity reduction of more than 50% is very subjective. Did this mean you had to be able to work less

Table 9: Fatigue in CFS (Holmes definition, 1988)	
1)	New onset
2)	No previous history of fatigue
3)	Does not resolve with bed rest
4)	Activity reduction greater than 50%
5)	Lasts longer than six months
6)	Exclude all other medical illnesses
7)	Exclude all psychiatric disorders

than half of the time? Or that you could only do 50% as much work as previously? Or that your leisure activities were reduced more than 50%? It was left to each physician and researcher to determine this, and each one did so differently, resulting in difficulty in deciding who really had this condition and how to study and treat it.

The notion that this fatigue had to be of new onset was also difficult to apply. We now know that Somatoneural Dysfuncton can be a lifelong disease that waxes and wanes based on a number of factors. It sounded like the patients of Dr. Holmes were suddenly struck with a crippling illness out of the blue and could not have overlapping features of other medical or psychiatric illnesses. In fact, though many patients with SND can point to an inciting event to their symptoms, the disorder generally progresses quite insidiously, thus making the course of illness vague rather than distinct. There is also a great degree of comorbidity with a variety of medical and psychiatric syndromes.

The associated clinical criteria were even harder to fulfill and were variable in degree and type. As you can see from Table 6, 8 of 14 of the "minor criteria" needed to be met for the diagnosis of CFS. They again added acute onset here for emphasis, I suppose, because if it was not of new onset, it couldn't be CFS according to their earlier statements.

Another problem was the attempt to turn CFS into an infectious illness. Six of the 14 criteria referred to symptoms of upper respiratory illness. You got a point for sore throat, painful lymph nodes, and low-grade fever and another point if the health care provider could document these symptoms. They had to split up these clinical findings because of the way patients presented. They had a lot of patients come to their office and say their throats were sore, that their lymph nodes were swollen, and that they had fevers, but on evaluation, none of these findings existed. Because they failed to understand why this happened, the authors had to structure the criteria with patient complaints and physical findings separately.

The inclusion of "generalized weakness" in the criteria was also quite controversial. In fact, true weakness is very rare in Somatoneural Dysfunction and should lead to a detailed search for other causes if it is really present. They were most likely mistaking fatigue for weakness, when in reality, the two symptoms are very different. Patients with SND have normal strength on maximal challenge testing, but are not able to sustain it for long and become unusually tired after the exertion.

Sleep disorders and impaired memory or concentration apply generally to most types of Somatoneural Dysfunction while the criteria of "migratory arthralgias" and "muscle aches" are sufficiently broad to apply to all types of SND as well. If a patient didn't have the infectious-type symptoms (numbers 1-6 in the Holmes criteria), they had to have all eight of the others to be classified as having chronic fatigue syndrome. This definition turned out to be too restrictive, selecting out only a small subset of patients, sometimes with widely variable clinical presentations.

Table 10: Minor Criteria of Holmes, 1988	
1)	Sore Throat
2)	Painful lymph nodes
3)	Low-grade fevers
4)	Documented low-grade fevers
5)	Documented nonexudative pharyngitis
6)	Documented tender lymph nodes
7)	Migratory arthralgias
8)	Impaired memory or concentration
9)	Unrefreshing sleep
10)	Muscle pain
11)	Generalized weakness
12)	Prolonged fatigue after exercise
13)	New generalized headaches
14)	New onset

In 1994, a revised definition was offered by Fukuda and colleagues at the Center for Disease Control in an attempt to rectify these problems. Their major criteria differed from Holmes in that it removed the need for activity reduction of greater than 50% and recognized that psychological comorbidity was a significant part of the syndrome. It should have been common sense that any patient who suffered more than six months of incapacitating fatigue along with all these other related symptoms would have an increased risk of depression and anxiety disorder.

The minor criteria put forth by the CDC had been whittled down to eight components, removing the need for documented fevers, lymph nodes, and exudative pharyngitis. This is fortunate because I have rarely heard of a patient to present with six months of fevers, lymph node swelling, and pus in the back of their throats. If a patient walks into my office with these symptoms, something very bad is going on (cancer, abscess) and it is not SND. They removed the criteria for low-grade fevers entirely and took out the weakness component. They additionally required only that four of the eight criteria be met.

Table 11: CDC Criteria for Chronic Fatigue Syndrome, 1994	
Major Criteria	**Minor Criteria (4 of 8)**
1) New onset	1) Sore throat
2) No previous history of fatigue	2) Painful lymph nodes
3) Does not resolve with bed rest	3) Generalized (new) headaches
4) Lasts longer than six months	4) Muscle pain
5) Exclude all other medical illnesses	5) Prolonged fatigue after exercise
6) Unrefreshing sleep	
7) Migratory arthralgias	
8) Impaired memory or concentration	

These criteria, in contrast to the Holmes definition of six years prior, have proved to be very broad. They still maintained, however, the link to infectious illness, mainly because they were established by infectious disease specialists! I believe that the patients they were studying were a mixed group of those with general Somatoneural Dysfunction and those with a subset-type of SND that would historically be called chronic fatigue syndrome. As we discuss CFS, we have to keep this in mind. Fortunately, the research on CFS has shed quite a bit of light on SND. I will explore some of the common issues as well as point out where chronic fatigue syndrome is unique.

Infections and Immune System Function

The Virus Question

The search for a viral cause of Somatoneural Dysfunction continues virtually unabated, costing millions each year in what is probably a futile endeavor. Why? Identification of a new virus responsible for chronic fatigue syndrome would be an earth-shattering discovery, worth fame and fortune to the researchers. A virus would make a much nicer target to direct our efforts against, like a common enemy. For the patients it would provide hope of specific treatments and preventative strategy, much like what has happened with the human immunodeficiency virus (HIV). Unfortunately, life in general, and medicine in particular does not work that way often enough and we are left with a complicated syndrome that involves virtually every major organ system in the body. Fighting a virus would be much simpler (and easier to explain to patients).

Certainly, investigators had reason to suspect an infectious source over the years, but with outbreaks and clusters of patients becoming less common and the syndrome spanning all types of people throughout the world, infection becomes less likely. The most likely culprit infection would certainly have been the always-elusive virus.

Some viral infections have the ability to cause an infection and lie dormant in our bodies, waiting to spring upon us again and cause recurrent symptoms. Viral particles or even intact virus can be isolated from blood or tissue decades after infection, such as the herpes simplex virus that causes cold sores. Other viruses, such as hepatitis B and C, can cause chronic infections as well. Of course, the human immuno-deficiency virus (HIV) is the most widely-studied chronic infection, causing its effects years and decades after initial contact.

The first virus that was implicated in chronic fatigue syndrome was the Epstein-Barr Virus (EBV), a member of the herpes virus family. It is the cause of infectious mononucleosis, or mono, the dreaded "kissing disease", an illness with the familiar features of low-grade fever, lymph node swelling, sore throat, and malaise. Studies done in the early 1980s revealed that as many as 90% of the patients affected with CFS had detectable antibodies to EBV. Subsequent studies, however, not only disproved a causal connection between EBV and CFS, but also discovered that nearly as many asymptomatic people without chronic fatigue syndrome (up to 95% in some areas) had detectable EBV antibodies as well (including this author).

Almost every time a new virus is discovered, attempts are made to link it to chronic fatigue syndrome, as was the case with newly detected herpes viruses 6, 7, and 8. Human herpes virus 6 (HHV-6) in particular was promising for a while, as it also was found in large numbers of chronic fatigue syndrome patients. However, HHV-6 was also found to be the virus responsible for roseola, an infection that virtually all Americans are exposed to by the age of four.

Another theory conceded that EBV and HHV-6 were found in most people, both those with chronic fatigue syndrome and those without it, but that the viruses somehow acted differently in the CFS patients. It is known that both viruses stay in patients for life and can be "reactivated" if the circumstances are right and cause further illness. The closely related varicella-zoster virus is the best known example of this process, causing chicken pox as the initial infection and herpes zoster ("shingles") if it becomes reactivated. Epstein-Barr Virus is associated with rare forms of lymphomas and tumors of the nasopharynx in certain ethnic populations, while HHV-6 can cause interstitial pneumonitis in bone marrow transplant patients who have suppressed immune systems (Levine, 1995).

Other viruses and bacterial infections have been loosely linked to Somatoneural Dysfunction, but the evidence is shaky at best. European studies have isolated a higher frequency of enteroviral DNA in the stool of patients with chronic fatigue syndrome and have attempted to link chronic coxsackie B virus infection to fibromyalgia (Bell, 1994). The rates of reactivation and even infection with these viruses is even less than for the herpesvirus group. One group of researchers reportedly found a certain gene sequence from human T-lymphotropic virus type 2 (HTLV-II) virus in CFS patients (Buchwald, 1996). This agent, a retrovirus similar to HIV, is responsible for cutaneous T-cell lymphoma and a spastic paralytic disease that occurs in Asia and the Caribbean. However, subsequent studies failed to document any connection or pattern in CFS and concluded that there was only a chance association in the initial study.

So, What is Going on With All These Viruses?

What all these researchers were finding was typically an increase in the antibody response to certain viral infections, the most widely studied being Epstein-Barr Virus. In some cases, like that of HHV-6, an increase in active replication of the virus was noted. It therefore appears that if a patient who has been previously infected with EBV gets chronic fatigue syndrome, the virus becomes more active. If the same patient has HHV-6 or coxsackie B virus, or varicella, or just about any other chronic viral infection, then that particular virus will become more active.

This should come as no surprise since we have known for years that viruses can reactivate under stressful conditions, such as the old cold sore virus herpes simplex. As you may recall from a few chapters ago, stress suppresses the immune system function. The stress can be medical (another illness or injury), physical (overwork and overexertion), or mental (loss of a loved one or financial strain).

It seems that in Somatoneural Dysfunction there are two abnormalities: 1) an immune system that is disordered and 2) an exaggerated susceptibility of the immune system to stress. Our immune system is like an army, protecting us from invaders and injury, but it has only so many resources at its disposal. The immune system also functions to keep chronic viral infections in check, but this taxes these resources. Devoting an immunologic brigade to keep an eye on a pesky herpes zoster virus hiding out in the nerve root of your thoracic dermatome occupies important cells and antibodies of the immune system.

If the troops from that brigade are called to fight off an upper respiratory infection or repair a broken ankle or even assist in coping with the loss of a loved one, the system is strained. As the suppressive function of the immune system is strained, the virus becomes more active, and shingles can develop if it "breaks loose". Other infections become more active and may initiate inflammatory responses as a second line of defense. These emergency mechanisms can make patients with Somatoneural Dysfunction feel a vague flulike-illness, occasionally even manifesting as fever, sore throat, or swollen lymph nodes. More often, patients with a persistently strained immune system and beleaguered inflammatory system just plain don't feel good. This is typically caused by release of cytokines such as IL-2 and TNF-α, which act to stimulate other areas of the immune system to work harder, but also tend to elevate body temperature and drain the body of energy.

Thus it is commonly accepted that the higher level of expression of viral DNA and antibody production is not due to clinical recurrence of infection with a virus, but is a marker of immune system activity in keeping these viruses in check.

We must keep in mind that it is not the virus itself that causes a fever, for example, but the body's reaction in fighting off the virus. People with suppressed immune systems, either from severe medical illness or from immune system suppression from strong medications (such as chemotherapy drugs), often show no signs of fever during infections.

On the other hand, fever may be caused by a number of non-infectious sources, such as tumors, rheumatologic diseases, damage to temperature-control centers in the brain, or just plain being out in the hot sun too long. It is the non-infectious activation of the immune system in SND that causes patients to feel feverish and generally yucky for long periods of time.

Immune System Dysfunction in Somatoneural Dysfunction

We can see some of findings of a strained immune system in the blood and tissues of patients with SND, but they are difficult to analyze and widely variable. The natural killer cell (NK) seems to be directly involved. This cell, the infantry of the immune system, acts to nonspecifically ward off infection, inflammation, and even tumor cells in some instances. Like any good soldier, the natural killer cell just goes where it is told and does its job. In chronic fatigue syndrome patients, however, there is a decreased activity of the NK cells, leading to a diminished ability to kill infecting organisms. There are also fewer cells around to begin with (Buchwald, 1996). Furthermore, stress inhibits NK cell activity, presumably through interactions between the brain and the immune system via signals sent by hormones such as neuropeptide Y, which has receptors on NK cells.

Cytokines are biochemicals in the body that signal other cells to perform a particular function. They are intricately involved in the immune response. In Somatoneural Dysfunction, studies have not been able to show consistent findings with regards to levels or activity of these agents. However, there are abnormalities in virtually every study. Interleukin-2 (IL-2) and tumor necrosis factor (two of the most important cytokines in the immune and inflammatory responses, as mentioned previously) have been studied extensively in different populations of chronic fatigue patients. Sometimes the levels are low, sometimes high, sometimes they don't work very well, and sometimes they are overzealous and work too hard. In nearly every case, however, there is some abnormality in cytokine function

A pattern did not appear initially from these studies. When you consider the orderliness that is typical of the immune system and its response, the pattern is actually the lack of a pattern! In Somatoneural Dysfunction, the tightly regulated system of immune function activation, regulation, and deactivation seems to be lost. When faced with the usual challenges of infection, stress, injury, and so on, the immune system of SND patients simply does not work right.

There is other evidence for immune system dysfunction in SND, but the evidence is not as well documented. There may be reduced proliferation of peripheral blood lymphocytes in response to stimulation, a decreased ability of lymphocytes and neutrophils to migrate to site of infection or inflammation, decreased wound healing, and an overall impaired effectiveness in destroying viral invaders. There is also probably a defect in the way the immune system responds to vaccinations and this may explain observations that patients with SND often become ill after receiving vaccines (Glaser, 1998).

Neuroendocrine Abnormalities in Somatoneural Dysfunction

We have arrived back at the hypothalamic-pituitary-adrenal axis (HPAA), that confusing system of hormones that leads from the brain to the adrenal glands and other hormone-producing organs via the pituitary gland. It appears that there are a number of abnormalities in the HPAA system in Somatoneural Dysfunction. Similar findings have been discovered in the subsets of fibromyalgia and chronic fatigue syndrome indicating again a shared pathology (Demitrack, 1994)).

Initial studies in the early 1990s showed a number of derangements in the HPAA including a lower baseline level of cortisol in the bloodstream , higher level of cortisol-binding globulin (CBG), and a normal adrenocortico-tropin hormone (ACTH) level. These were found mainly in evening samples. Normally, there is peak cortisol release in the morning, production of several spurts of cortisol during the day, and a lower level at night. This corresponds to a "circadian rhythm" which is commonly seen in bodily systems involved in sleep-wake cycles and a multitude of other functions. Generally, our bodies need more active functions during the day and more restorative functions at night.

Overall there was a reduced total cortisol as measured by a 24-hour collection of urine along with a normal peak level of cortisol in the morning. If we put this together, our heads tend to hurt. However, if we call upon some very smart people in long white coats to explain this to us, things become a little clearer. They tell me this means that there is a dysregulation in the brain and pituitary control of cortisol secretion because, in the presence of lower cortisol levels, there should be increased release of ACTH to compensate. Apparently this regulatory response is blunted in patients with Somatoneural Dysfunction.

Investigators found that giving CRH resulted in a reduced response and giving ACTH spurred an exaggerated response. It would appear again that the primary disorder in the HPAA in patients with Somatoneural Dysfunction is dysregulation. The system functions correctly under normal circumstances, but doesn't function the way it should when faced with stress. Normal ACTH responsiveness to stressful situations is impaired, leading to increased sensitivity of the pituitary and adrenals. This is another reason why the deficits in this syndrome have proven so elusive; patients feel normal and function normally until enough stress impacts on the system so that it can no longer compensate.

The thyroid may also play a role in chronic fatigue syndrome and Somatoneural Dysfunction. Thyroid function has generally been seen as normal in SND and related syndromes, however, there seems to be a significant overlap in SND patients and those that have been previously diagnosed as having "subclinical hypothyroidism". As mentioned earlier, patients with this problem have elevated levels of TSH, but normal free thyroid hormone. They also typically have problems with chronic fatigue. Subclinical hypothyroidism may also be asymptomatic, but may be a risk factor for SND, or simply a manifestation to the decreased overall metabolic response in SND.

Since the thyroid is partly responsible for metabolism, patients with SND may need higher levels of thyroid hormone in an attempt to compensate for some of the deficits in metabolic function. It is easy to see the theory behind this when you consider that the "normal" range of thyroid hormone is from 4.0 to 12.0, encompassing a 200% variation. What is typically a normal level of thyroid function is may simply not be enough to maintain proper metabolic activity in Somatoneural Dysfunction.

Summary

These pathophysiological changes in the endocrine and immune systems lead to symptoms in two basic ways.

1) Cytokine activation: the overexpression and dysregulation of inflammatory mediators of the immune system contribute to generalized fatigue, muscle and joint pains, and headaches. The mechanism and symptom complex is very similar to the way a person feels when suffering from a viral infection, just without the virus.

2) Dysruption of homeostatic functions of the endocrine system: abnormal regulation of the thyroid, pituitary, and adrenal systems leads to increased activation of sympathetic nerves. This increases central nervous system sensitivity to peripheral sensory stimuli and the detrimental impact of stress.

Reminders:

Cytokine: chemical that is really a type of hormone that acts to signal a cell to do something, usually to start or stop doing something

Homeostasis: the process of metabolic activity in the body that keeps things orderly and running properly

Fibromyalgia

Definition

Fibromyalgia was originally characterized by the American College of Rheumatology in 1990 to describe a fairly common condition that had widespread pain as an identifying feature without obvious physical findings. The World Health Organization followed suit and recognized fibromyalgia as a distinct disease in 1992. The guidelines proposed by the ACR are seen on the next page in table 11.

By itself, fibromyalgia is said to affect 7 to 10 million Americans and many millions more throughout the world. This may amount to up to 2% of the population at any given time. The incidence increases with age, although the average age of onset is between 29 and 37 years of age (Wolfe, 1995). Women account for nearly 85% of fibromyalgia patients, although the incidence of the disorder among male patients appears to be increasing.

The pain in fibromyalgia is characteristically scattered, and the patterns described below are a general guideline. The discomfort is often described as continuous, deep, and aching and may radiate diffusely along the lines of muscle or nerve. Typically, the pain in fibromyalgia is better with sustained exercise and worse with rest, although the fatigue experienced after exertion may be overwhelming at times. This usually is enough to differentiate fibromyalgia from advanced rheumatic conditions or osteoarthritis where stiffness with disuse or pain worsening with activity are common features.

Unfortunately, when first beginning to exercise, the patient with fibromyalgia experiences an increase in pain. This deters them from continuing to exercise and the potential benefit from continued physical conditioning is never realized. This is true of many other muscle and tendon conditions, such as plantar fasciitis (heel spur syndrome) where the feet can be excruciatingly painful when first walking on them. This pain also characteristically lessens with continued walking.

Many other symptoms have been linked with fibromyalgia, including nonrestorative sleep, fatigue, and morning achiness (Ang, 1999). Functional disability, psychological distress, irritable bowel syndrome, headache, diffuse parasthesia, and a subjective feeling of swelling in the limbs may also occur. There is obviously significant overlap between fibromyalgia and the other disorders listed here, thus it merits inclusion as a subtype of Somatoneural Dysfunction. Perhaps the majority of SND patients have fibromyalgia at some time in their life or another. If the symptoms are sustained and severe, they come for medical attention, but if they are not, often the patients simply go about life as best they can. Thus there is a wide difference in manifestation of fibromyalgia from mild, intermittent cases, to severe, almost disabling ones.

Table 12: ACR Criteria for Classification of Fibromyalgia

1.   History of widespread pain (presenting at all the following sites):
•   Right and Left side of the body (including shoulders and buttocks)
•   Above and below the waist
•   In axial skeleton (cervical spine or anterior chest, thoracic spine or low back

2.   Pain on digital palpation (performed with about 4 kg of force) in 11 of 18 sites (bilateral points at each site)
•   Occiput (at suboccipetal muscle insertion)
•   Low cevical (at anterior intertransverse spaces of C5-C7)
•   Supraspinatus (above scapula, near medial border of spine)
•   Second rib (at second costochondral junctions, just beside junctions on the upper surfaces)
•   Lateral epicondyle (2 cm distal to the epicondyles)
•   Gluteal (upper outer quadrants of the buttocks)
•   Greater trochanter (posterior to trochanteric prominance)
•   Knee (at medial fat pad proximal to the joint line)

Classification of Fibromyalgia

Although fibromyalgia is distinguished by the prominence of pain, sleep disturbance and central nervous system sensitization are central to its pathogenesis. The presence of autonomic dysfunction, decreased efficiency of the stress response and decreased function of the hypothalamic-pituitary-adrenal axis are characteristic of fibromyalgia and Somatoneural Dysfunction in general. If we wanted to provide a narrower classification we could call this "Somatoneural Dysfunction-Pain Predominant" to differentiate it from chronic fatigue syndrome, which could then be called "Somatoneural Dysfunction-Fatigue Predominant". I like to keep things simple though, and the striking similarities among all the SND subtypes lend themselves most easily to classification as a single entity.

Pain in Fibromyalgia

The type and extent of pain in fibromyalgia is its most distinguishing feature, but really shares a common theme with Somatoneural Dysfunction; that of dysregulation or overactivity of a normal bodily function. Patients with fibromyalgia have a lowered threshold to pain, which is one of the body's strongest protective mechanisms. This has been confirmed in a number of studies using pressure devices (Mikkelsson, 1992). Interestingly, most fibromyalgia patients actually think that they have an unusually high pain threshold. This is likely to be a part of the abnormal way sensory information about pain is processed and interpreted by the brain in fibromyalgia.

Pain in fibromyalgia is "all over" and often involves, not only joints and muscles, but also headache, nerve-type pain and parasthesias, bladder and bowel pain, and cramping. Tender point sensitivity is common, but by no means always present, and the distribution of painful sites corresponds to minor aches and pains of everyday life in patients without fibromyalgia (Winfield, 1999).

The key here is to learn why these "normal" aches and pains result in exhaustive, debilitating pain perception in fibromyalgia patients.

> "These patients are just wimps!"—second-year medical student
> "They're all depressed"—hematology fellow
> "They only need to get their minds off it"—medical attending

Unfortunately, quotes and attitudes such as these from the medical profession have hindered research into fibromyalgia and alienated patients who need to work very closely with their physicians. Biological discoveries over the last two decades, however, have allowed us to determine that there really is significant underlying pathology and put much of the misunderstanding to rest.

Physiological Abnormalities in Pain Processing

Much the same way that diabetics cannot efficiently process sugar, fibromyalgia patients cannot effectively process pain. There appears to be not only a decreased threshold for pain tolerance, but also in pain discrimination where typically non-painful stimuli (such as pressure, warmth, or cold) are perceived as painful. There have been at least a dozen well designed, carefully controlled, randomized clinical trials which have proved this (see the excellent article by Winfield to review them), but I have a very hard time convincing my patients of this.

> "I took a bayonet in the back of my head during WWII, and bit on a bullet while they stitched me up!"

> "I gave birth to a 12-pound baby, without pain medicine...C-section!"

I hear these stories from fibromyalgia patients when I tell them of their decreased pain tolerance and I am sure they are true. There is a difference, however, between tender-point pain and the acute pain that comes from a sharp knife in the head. As you might recall from chapter 2 (you can look it up if you want, I'll wait!), there is a neurologic distinction between acute and chronic pain. While a patient with fibromyalgia may think nothing of a knife wound, they may be nearly crippled by lingering pain from a mildly sprained ankle. Occasionally, the perception of both acute and chronic pain may be affected, but more often the disease process involves chronic pain alone. The biologic response to pressure measured by a dolorimeter more closely resembles chronic pain than acute.

Several abnormalities in the pathways of pain perception by the nervous system have been identified in fibromyalgia. Increased levels of substance P, the neurotransmitter involved in processing and sending painful signals to the brain, has been found in peripheral nerves and in cerebrospinal fluid. This leads to hyperexcitability of cells in the nervous system that receive painful stimuli, causing them to be very sensitive.

Serum levels of serotonin are significantly lower than normal in patients with fibromyalgia (Yunus, 1992). Although difficult to measure and data are conflicting, is it suspected that levels of serotonin in brain tissue are also decreased. Depletion of serotonin leads to decrease in NREM sleep, increased awareness of somatic sensation, and increased perception of pain (McCain, 1994). It also causes depression.

Brand new studies by Larson, Russell, and others have also shown a decrease in serotonin and an increase in excitatory pain neurotransmitters in the cerebrospinal fluid of patients with fibromyalgia (Larson, 2000). This practically confirms theories that suggest a central nervous system abnormality as central to the pathogenesis of fibromyalgia and SND.

A relatively new and potentially exciting area of interest in fibromyalgia and pain research is the NMDA receptor. The N-methyl-D-aspartic acid (NMDA) receptors are found on neurons that respond to painful stimuli. They are activated by excitatory neurotransmitters (mainly glutamine and asparagine, for those keeping score) released by pain fibers from the peripheral nervous system. Once activated, these receptors cause the release of good old substance P. It stands to reason that overexcitation of NMDA receptors may exist in fibromyalgia, since that would explain the high levels of substance P and hypersensitivity to pain.

One very small study assessed the efficacy of treating fibromyalgia patients with an NMDA-receptor blocker (ketamine). The majority of the patients improved, but side effects were significant (Sorensen, 1997). More research needs to be done in this area to determine the benefits of modulating the NMDA-receptor. Several pharmaceutical companies are working on drugs that block the receptor to act as a general pain reliever at the moment.

There appears to also be a decrease in blood flow and in functional activity in the thalamus and caudate nucleus in the brain. These areas are involved in the inhibition of pain and decreased blood flow seems to indicate decreased pain tolerance. Fibromyalgia patients thus have two abnormalities in the control of pain that lead to decreased tolerance: an increase in the sensitivity to pain and a decrease in the body's natural ability to defend against painful stimuli.

Pain (nociception) should only occur at times of tissue injury (from pressure, trauma, inflammation, etc), but in fibromyalgia there is pain perception without tissue injury. However, the brain and central nervous system respond in exactly the same way they do during tissue injury as reflected by the above studies. In other words, fibro patients have the same pattern of neurochemical response and brain activity as other patients with chronic pain such as rheumatoid arthritis, without any obvious source of pain.

Predisposition to Pain in Fibromyalgia

Some patients have a particular susceptibility to the pain dys-regulation that occurs in fibromyalgia. There seems to be a genetic component, as relatives of patients with fibromyalgia have a greater likelihood of having impaired pain tolerance in general as well as having fibromyalgia themselves (Buskila, 1997). Peak onset of fibromyalgia occurs between the ages of 30-50, although it certainly can occur in children or the elderly. This is generally true of most neurologic and rheumatic disorders and is probably nothing more than a timing effect where the nervous system response to pain starts to become dysfunctional.

The stress response of the HPAA is involved in pain tolerance and is also abnormal in fibromyalgia. The HPAA contributes heavily to the control of pain through mechanisms designed to release endogenous opioids (such as endorphins and enkephalins) in order to diminish pain at the level of the spinal cord, at nerve endings, and in painful tissue directly. Chronic stress leads to HPAA suppression and decrease function of this natural pain defense system.

The contribution of neurally-mediated hypotension to altered pain perception should not be overlooked either. Patients who had temporomendibular dysfunction (TMD or TMJ more commonly) and low blood pressure had more pain than those with high blood pressure (Maixner, 1997). This initial study was reproduced in normal subjects with similar results (Angrilli, 1997). The result appeared to be much more dramatic in chronic, aching types of pain than in acute pains from heat or lack of blood flow. This supports a great deal of evidence that low blood pressure suppresses the activation of arterial pressure receptors that decrease pain threshold and tolerance and can lead to increased anxiety (Sheffield, 1994). This is an example of the body's protective response to encourage maintenance of adequate blood pressure in order to keep blood flowing to important organs and tissues. The effect seems to level off at the upper limits of normal blood pressure because it is no longer necessary for protection.

Pain sensation is also increased by relative inactivity and decreased physical fitness. This relationship has been established long ago in patients with rheumatoid and osteoarthritis and holds true as well for fibromyalgia and Somatoneural Dysfunction. I like to refer to this as "The Vicious Spiral" and really reflects common sense. If you have a lot of pain and you are tired all the time, you will find it difficult to exercise and keep well conditioned. Deconditioning in turn will lead to decreased muscle mass, thinning of the bones, and deterioration of connective tissue in tendons and ligaments. This all combines increased susceptibility to further pain and the spiral goes down even further.

Figure 4: The Spiral

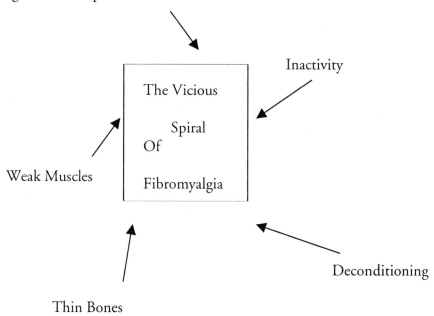

Gender also plays a determining role in fibromyalgia. Women are several times more likely than men to have abnormal pain perception. This is due to a number of factors listed in Table 13 below, but the general rationale for this increased sensitivity in females is simply an increased protective response. Let's face it guys, in the survival of the species, women are way more important than men. Because their ability to bear and nurture children leaves them more vulnerable than men (decreased muscle mass, etc), women developed some protective mechanisms. These include a heightened response to pain, as well as something called "women's intuition", which is a whole other topic entirely.

Table 13: Reasons Why Women Are More Sensitive to Pain	
1) Input to the central nervous system	enhanced through regulatory hormone fluctuation during the menstrual cycle
2) CNS pain processing	hormone modulation of pain regulation, stress-response to pain, and opioid receptors
3) Emotional responses	higher rate of anxiety and depressive disorders
4) Coping strategies	increased maladaptive behavior in response to pain
5) Peripheral responses	stress and pain less likely to induce HPAA responses

Interestingly, there also appears to be an accessory "estrogen-dependent" pathway involved in the perception of pain. This pathway seems to be independent of and inhibitory to pathways involving endorphins and the NMDA-receptor cascade (Touchette, 1993). How this system relates to pain in fibromyalgia and whether it explains why women are more susceptible to fibromyalgia remains to be seen.

Finally, decreased sleep plays a role in pain defense:

1) physically via recovery of muscle and joint function
2) neurologically by selective release of serotonin and endorphins, and
3) psychologically through dream mechanisms of coping.

The poor sleep patterns seen in fibromyalgia thus contribute to the initiation of and maintenance of these specific patterns of pain. Sleep disturbances will be discussed in more detail a bit later. In addition, the psychological aspects of pain perception and defense are also extremely important. They will be discussed soon as well.

Other Abnormalities in Fibromyalgia: The Stress Response

Fibromyalgia shares many characteristics of an abnormal stress response with chronic fatigue syndrome. It was this striking similarity that first led me to research common pathways in the two disorders and investigate the many common threads. The abnormalities in the hypothalamic-pituitary-adrenal axis seen in chronic fatigue syndrome may also be present in fibromyalgia, again suggesting a common pathophysiology. Similarly, deficiencies in central nervous system serotonin regulation of the stress response also contribute to the abnormal stress response. This explains why stress, either physical or psychological, often causes symptoms of fibromyalgia to flare up.

Many patients with Somatoneural Dysfunction, particularly fibromyalgia, point to a specific event as inciting their illness. For some this is a viral or bacterial infection, leading researchers to initially speculate on an infectious cause similar to the story for chronic fatigue syndrome. For others, trauma (such as whiplash from a minor motor vehicle accident) seems to trigger the syndrome.

This syndrome of "reactive" or "posttraumatic" fibromyalgia has garnered a lot of negative press recently. This appears to be related mainly to litigation claims or requests for disability and has been generalized to a certain extent to fibromyalgia patients as a whole. There is likely a certain "central sensitization" that occurs in patients with Somatoneural Dysfunction. This process reflects repeated dysregulated responses to stressful events, including injury, illness, or psychological trauma.

I know that if my patients with SND get in a car accident and suffer a whiplash-type injury, they will encounter a specific set of problems related to pain control and rehabilitation due to their disorder. The distinction comes from the symptomatology expressed by SND patients, who most often have a flare of their syndrome as a whole and not just from the injury.

For example, a patient with SND/fibromyalgia suffers a knee sprain in a rollerblading fall. Left untreated or improperly treated, he may have worsening fatigue, sleeplessness, and bowel irritability. The knee pain itself may last a bit longer without effective treatment, but generally responds to local care, anti-inflammatories, and physical therapy just as well as the knee of a patient without SND.

If a similar patient continues to have debilitating knee pain after appropriate time and effective treatment, then it is likely something else is contributing to the problem. They may have complex regional pain syndrome (reflex sympathetic dystrophy or causalgia), an injury and inflammation of associated nerves, which may be long lasting and refractory to treatment. Other types of nerve or tissue damage may occur and should be sought out. Finally, some patients may be malingering or faking their injury for financial gain. These patients are quite rare, but unfortunately, have made many medical practitioners leery of patients with chronic pain syndromes.

Personally, I believe that disability claims by patients with Somatoneural Dysfunction are often detrimental to the patient's recovery. As we shall discuss in the next book, there are multiple effective options for treatment of

SND and requests for disability should be viewed as a failure of treatment and a sign of "giving up". Fortunately, I my experience, very few SND patients reach this stage and most are able to continue productive lives despite their chronic illness. It may, however, be reasonable to obtain disability in severe cases requiring intensive treatment programs. This temporary disability time, maybe 6-12 months, can then be used to treat the illness.

That is not to say that fibromyalgia cannot be progressive and disabling. If left untreated, or if treatment programs are not followed, fibromyalgia and Somatoneural Dysfunction in general can be quite disabling. This is most often seen when the recurrent cycle of pain and inactivity leads to irreversible muscle and joint atrophy and myofascial contracture.

I view this as similar to the natural history of diabetes and hypertension. With proper diet, exercise, and medication, diabetes and hypertension should not adversely affect a patient's health over the course of their life. However, if not managed adequately, theses conditions can lead to heart attacks, stroke, blindness, amputation, and renal failure. For fibromyalgia patients, treatment is just as crucial.

Multiple Chemical Sensitivity Syndrome

Multiple chemical sensitivity (MCS) has been described under various names since the 1940s and is characterized by a wide variety of symptoms attributed by the patient to allergic or toxic exposure to things in the environment. Most commonly, these environmental exposures are man-made chemicals used in the workplace and can range from perfumes to solvents to cleaning agents. No direct evidence has been discovered that explains a connection between such exposures, calling into question whether or not the syndrome exists. Comments by the American Medical Association, 1992:

> "No evidence based on well-controlled clinical trials
> is available that supports a cause-and-effect relation-

ship between exposure to very low levels of substances and the myriad symptoms reported by clinical ecologists to result from such exposures…Until such accurate, reproducible, and well-controlled studies are available, the American Medical Association Council on Scientific Affairs believes that multiple chemical sensitivity should not be considered a recognized clinical syndrome"

"[MCS] has been rejected as an established organic disease by the American Academy of Allergy and Immunology, the American Medical Association, the California Medical Association, the American College of Physicians, and the International Society of Regulatory Toxicology and Pharmacology. It may be the only ailment in existence in which the patient defines both the cause and the manifestations of his own condition. Despite this, it has achieved credibility in workmen's compensation claims, tort liability, and regulatory actions"

—Gots, 1992

It would thus appear that the medical establishment doesn't think much of MCS. However, if we reconsider the fact that similar statements were made about fibromyalgia or chronic fatigue syndrome up until the last few years, we may want to take a closer look at this syndrome. Part of the suspiciousness comes from fact that most of these cases involve work-related incidents. There have been a few highly publicized cases (the worker on disability for back pain caught on videotape building a wall for his garden lifting sixty pound blocks of concrete, for example), which have resulted in extreme vigilance by occupational medicine to guard against fraud and abuse.

Therefore, anything related to worker's compensation or disability claims is held under close scrutiny. I have a diabetic patient who was a mail carrier despite his open-heart bypass, three heart attacks, insulin coma, and amputation of his left foot. When he had to have his right foot amputated because of severe peripheral vascular disease and gangrene I convinced him to apply for disability. After three denials and four appeals, including one accompanied by photographs of his open wounds, the disability bureau finally determined that being a mail carrier wasn't a good line of work for someone without any feet! So you can easily imagine what a patient must face to claim disability from a disorder without any known medical basis.

Thus, the pendulum has swung too far to the other end of the spectrum with the medical profession claiming that multiple chemical sensitivity doesn't exist as a defense against disability claims. The true effect of MCS lies, predictably, somewhere in the middle. I believe it does exist as an oversensitivity to chemical toxins or allergens much the same way fibromyalgia patients are oversensitized to pain and chronic fatigue syndrome sufferers are oversensitized to fatigue. None of these syndromes should be disabling, however, with proper education, understanding, and treatment.

The most widely accepted definition of MCS has been proposed by Cullen (1995).

Table 14: Cullen's Definition of Multiple Chemical Sensitivity

1) The syndrome is acquired by a documentable environmental exposure that may have caused objective evidence of health effects.

2) The symptoms are referable to multiple organ systems and vary predictably in response to environmental stimuli.

3) The symptoms occur in relation to measurable levels of chemicals, but the levels are below those known to cause harm to health no objective evidence of organ damage can be found

This definition does not rely on a proposed mechanism of disease or on specific symptoms due to the wide variation in different patients.

Symptoms

Symptoms in MCS generally fall into one of three categories (central nervous system, respiratory, or gastrointestinal), although virtually any symptom may be seen. The severity can range from mild to incapacitating. Often, a single large exposure triggers the symptoms, which then occur at low-level exposures that may have even been well tolerated previously.

Central nervous system symptoms include fatigue, difficulty concentrating, memory loss, headache, dizziness, weakness, and depression. This sounds an awful lot like what we've already been discussing, doesn't it? Gastrointestinal effects most commonly include nausea, heartburn and esophageal reflux, and diarrhea, which may be attributable to irritable bowel. Upper respiratory symptoms are mostly irritative and may comprise nasal stuffiness or runniness, dry cough, excess mucous production, burning or stinging eyes, tearing, wheezing, or shortness of breath.

Despite the fact that the majority of the cases of MCS are initiated by workplace environmental exposures, the symptoms cause dramatic effects on patients' lives. One occupational medicine study showed that 77% of patients with MCS left their jobs, while over 80% limited contact with friends, limited travel, and stopped activities outside the home (Lax, 1995). Drastic effects were also seen on personal care and home routines as patients sought to limit their exposure to any chemical in their environment. Certainly, anxiety and other psychiatric factors contributed to these activities, but were not the inciting event.

Possible Mechanisms of Disease

The most obvious possible causes of MCS are environmental allergy or cumulative toxin exposure. Extensive studies done, however, in search of immunologic or toxic effects in patients have proven fruitless. Tests of allergic reactivity failed to show any difference between patients with MCS and those without (Kehrl, 1997). Other studies have looked at toxicologic effect from various environmental factors in MCS patients, but found none. Some claim that MCS is a manifestation of a "homeopathy", where patients have clinical symptoms from exposure to levels of chemicals or allergens too low to detect pathologic changes. This is kind of like saying that the Easter Bunny causes MCS; you can't see him, you can't prove he's there, no one's ever proven he's there, but the Easter eggs are all painted so he must exist.

Easter bunnies notwithstanding, another theory of MCS seems to fit in nicely with the general premise of Somatoneural Dysfunction. It is possible that affected people develop increasing sensitization to adverse effects of chemical exposures. Little by little, these exposures build to levels where clinical responses are seen. They occur in patients who are susceptible due to dysregulation in their immune responses or in their bodies' natural defense to certain toxins. Continued exposures then overwhelm the system and trigger MCS.

This theory is supported by animal studies that have shown the effects of a "kindling" or sensitization response that occurs when repeated low-level chemical or electrical exposure is applied. This repeated exposure sets up a change in receptor sensitivity so that it responds to lower and lower levels of exposure (Barr, 1997). This has not, however, been shown to occur in humans (such trials would be highly unethical), nor at the low doses reported to cause MCS, so this theory too remains speculative.

Psychiatric factors may certainly play a role in the development of MCS, similar to the way they interplay with the biological phenomena occurring in fibromyalgia or chronic fatigue syndrome. MCS patients are very likely to suffer from depression, anxiety disorder, panic attacks, post-traumatic stress disorder, and somatization disorder. Like other types of SND, it is more likely that MCS and psychiatric effects seen in patients share a common causal relationship rather than simply one causing the other.

Table 15: Principles of Management of MCS Syndrome	
Goals	Avoid
Maximize rehabilitation	Unproven therapies
Control (not cure) symptoms	Antifungal treatment for candidiasis
Treat accompanying psychiatric and medical illness	Rotating diets
Activity as tolerated	Extreme avoidance of chemicals
Desensitization to provocative agents	Social isolation
Relaxation exercises	
Reassurance that autonomic symptoms are not dangerous	
	(Dietert, 1997)

As you can see, the best way to treat MCS is with understanding and education. Decreasing stress levels and accompanying symptoms of depression and anxiety is central to the treatment plan, as is avoiding potentially harmful or unproven remedies. The only part of the treatment program that is truly unique to MCS is desensitization to provocative agents. This is similar to the way allergists treat other environmental allergies. For example, if exposure to an offending chemical is unavoidable, patients may desensitize themselves by gradually increasing their exposure over time. This assumes, of course, that the chemical is proven to hold no inherent danger. Other treatment avenues follow those of Somatoneural Dysfunction in general.

Neurally-Mediated Hypotension

Chronic fatigue and chronic fatigue syndrome has been linked with abnormal changes in blood pressure in recent years. Studies began to accumulate over the past decade that linked chronic hypotension with fatigue. A British study of over ten thousand patients concluded that a lower systolic blood pressure reading was associated with complaints of dizziness, tiredness, and muscle aches and pains sounding similar to those seen frequently in Somatoneural Dysfunction (Rowe, 1998)

Orthostatic hypotension is a disorder of the regulation of blood pressure by the autonomic nervous system. When you stand up from a seated or supine position, your body must re-equilibrate to compensate for the change in pressure caused by gravity. If this system doesn't work right, all the blood pools in your legs, none reaches your brain, and you suddenly have a great desire to run for Congress. No, actually, you feel dizzy, lightheaded, and like you're going to pass out. Wait a minute, that is like being in congress after all…

Another study described chronic fatigue in patients whose blood pressure fell more than 30 mmHg systolic within 5 minutes of standing upright. These patients too had feelings of lightheadedness, but also noted problems thinking and concentrating, tremulousness, and anxiety. Patients with dramatic orthostasis may pass out entirely.

The usual increase in blood flow to the brain is mediated by the vagus nerve, predominantly by altering release of norepinephrine and epinephrine. Failure to do so can result in "vasodepressor syncope" which results in fainting. Vessels in the limbs and muscles dilate and shunt the blood away from the brain where it would be (somewhat) more useful. The medulla is the part of the brain that receives and sends signals from the vagus nerve and usually acts to regulate this blood flow.

This system developed in humans as another protective response to allow more blood to flow to the muscles for the fight or flight mechanism. When it becomes oversensitive or overactive, fainting may occur. This can be seen with strong emotion (fright, anger, sadness), particularly in the setting of hot, crowded rooms, alcohol consumption, tiredness, or hunger. All of these conditions favor dilation of the blood vessels. The feeling of faintness can also occur with pain or strenuous physical exertion.

Types of fainting, or syncope, are varied. Neurocardiogenic syncope occurs when the receptors that control volume of output from the heart are dysregulated. Some patients may develop syncope with pressure on the neck if the carotid sinus receptors are sensitive, while others may be sensitive to the pressure changes within the body that occur with urination, defecation, breath-holding, or strenuous exercise.

True orthostatic hypotension occurs without a protective increase in heart rate and is mediated predominantly by a defect in the way the receptors in the blood vessels react to changes and position. Patients with neurally-mediated hypotension (NMH) have both a defect in these receptors and abnormal communication with the central nervous system via the vagus nerve.

Perhaps the first described case of this phenomenon occurred in 1932 in Britain by Sir Thomas Lewis. He described a soldier with a history of exhaustion after exercise and fainting while on duty. The soldier fainted after having his blood drawn and was found to have a very low blood pressure. He became severely fatigued and anxious for the next few days, showing that prolonged symptoms could occur after a single episode of fainting (Lewis, 1932).

Studies have shown that patients with this syndrome are more frequently female and most likely between the ages of 20 and 50. It may run in families and often occurs after an acute infectious illness. It is commonly accompanied by panic attacks. Patients may have a lower resting blood pressure, thus making them more susceptible. There is obviously a significant overlap between neurally-medicated hypotension and other types of Somatoneural Dysfunction.

Patients with NMH don't actually faint often, but they may have a chronically abnormal hypotensive response to exertion, similar to that seen in chronic fatigue syndrome. This response results in decreased functioning of the normal compensatory system and can lead to a variety of symptoms. These include a feeling of "fogginess" that may be continuous or intermittent, deterioration in memory and concentration, lightheadedness, fatigue, shakiness, and soft tissue swelling of the feet and ankles (Low, 1995). These responses can be documented by testing on a tilt-table that provides information about how the system reacts to different positions. In Somatoneural Dysfunction there may be a low-level defect in the system that may not show up as obviously on testing.

This abnormal autonomic nervous system response or dysautonomia is also commonly seen in fibromyalgia and chronic fatigue syndrome as well. Low levels of neuropeptide Y (NPY) have been shown in a number of patients with Somatoneural Dysfunction. NPY is found with norepinephrine at nerve terminals and plays an important role in function of the stress response by the hypothalamic-pituitary-adrenal axis and maintaining capillary blood flow. Inability of the capillaries to correct for position changes results in relative hypotension and decreased blood flow to the brain (Clauw, 1995).

Another important stress hormone is arginine vasopressin (AVP). This hormone, also called antidiuretic hormone or ADH (by people like me who find this easier to remember), is actually part of a separate parallel system from the HPAA. It is made in the hypothalamus (the parvocellular division of the paramedian nucleus, for those who are keeping score at home) and stored in the posterior part of the pituitary (also called the neurohypophysis). For some reason, many of these things have two or more names, which is why I have generally stayed out of research and concentrated on caring for patients. They, for the most part, only have one or two names.

Antidiuretic hormone is stored in the pituitary, unlike the other pituitary hormones, which are made there. The brain manages fluid volume very closely because it allows humans to live on dry land, or so my old Earth Science teacher told me. It does this in two ways; by thirst, which regulates the amount of fluid coming in, and by ADH, which acts in the kidney to regulate the amount of fluid going out.

ADH also acts to directly stimulate ACTH release. ACTH is the hormone most responsible for activating cortisol from the adrenal glands. In response to stress, ADH greatly magnifies the ability of CRH (corticotropin releasing hormone, from the brain) to release ACTH and thus increases circulating levels of cortisol. Abnormal sensitivity of this "volume-control" system may also contribute to defective regulation of blood pressure and thus, neurally-mediated hypotension.

Whether or not this is a distinct syndrome or merely a component of some cases of Somatoneural Dysfunction remains to be more firmly established. In any event, significant symptoms of lightheadedness, dizziness, or fainting in a patient with SND should raise consideration of neurally-mediated hypotension once other causes have been ruled out. I have rarely found it necessary to perform detailed tilt-table testing, usually only in cases where prolonged medication therapy is contemplated to alleviate symptoms.

Treatment is first aimed at adjusting the diet to enhance sodium retention and increasing physical activity to strengthen the cardiovascular system. If this conservative approach is not effective, inotropic medications can be used. These agents enhance blood pressure and limit the fall in pressure that occurs with a change in position. Unfortunately, as we will see a bit later, these medications also have many unwanted side effects.

Irritable Bowel Syndrome

Irritable bowel syndrome (IBS) is an extremely common, worldwide disorder of altered bowel function. A prevalence of 15% to 20% is consistent in such widely varied geographical and ethnic groups as China and the U.S. Less than half of the patients with IBS ever seek medical advice unless they also suffer from other symptoms of SND. As many as 50% of patients referred to gastroenterology specialists have IBS (Lynn, 1995).

Irritable bowel syndrome may appear on its own or in association with other subtypes of Somatoneural Dysfunction, most commonly Chronic Fatigue Syndrome and Fibromyalgia. Symptoms tend to be somewhat worse if these disorders coexist.

The official diagnostic criteria for irritable bowel syndrome can be found in the Table 12, but I prefer to use the Manning Criteria. These six symptoms have been found to predict IBS symptoms in the setting of SND and include:

1) Pain relief with bowel action
2) More frequent stools with the onset of pain
3) Looser stools with the onset of pain
4) Passage of mucus
5) Sensation of incomplete evacuation
6) Abdominal distention as evidenced by tight clothing or visible appearance (Lynn, 1995)

The more of these symptoms that are present, the greater likelihood of IBS. Symptoms of gastroespohageal reflux are common and fatigue, muscle aches, poor sleep, and other cardinal manifestations of SND are likely to be present as well. It has always been assumed that IBS is a distinct disorder related to abnormal gastrointestinal motility, but I believe it is another manifestation of SND.

Table 16: Diagnostic Criteria for Irritable Bowel Syndrome

At least three months of continuous or recurrent symptoms
Abdominal pain or discomfort that is:
- relieved with defecation,
- associated with a change in frequency of stool, or
- associated with a change in consistency of stool
and
Two or more of the following, at least 25% of the time
- altered stool frequency (more than 3 per day or less than 3 per week)
- altered stool form (hard/loose/watery)
- altered stool passage (straining/urgency/incomplete evacuation)
- passage of mucus
- feeling of bloating or abdominal distention

(Boyce, 2000)

Irritable bowel syndrome has often been called "functional bowel disease" because it was difficult to find a pathological defect in such patients. The fact that stress often worsened the symptoms of IBS strengthened the belief that the disorder was psychosomatic. However, like other aspects of SND, there seems to be a hypersensitivity of the normally functioning bowel in IBS.

The process of getting food from the lips to the anus is extraordinary complex. It is a controlled by a complicated neurological and musculoskeletal process that is influenced by both hormonal and psychological factors. There are four main presentations of IBS:

1) Diarrhea predominant
2) Constipation predominant
3) Alternating diarrhea and constipation
4) Pain predominant

Patients may fit mainly into one category or vary between categories periodically. They may also have a combination of features. Whatever the presentation, however, the root of the problem in IBS seems to go along with the common theme of Somatoneural Dysfunction. There appears again to be a specific biological system under control of a sensitive and abnormally responsive central nervous system.

Normal Bowel Function

Food is moved from the mouth to the anus mainly by the process of peristalsis. This is the process of smooth muscle contraction that acts to squeeze the food through roughly thirty feet of intestines to arrive at the rectum. These contractions come in waves, both a high frequency, low power baseline wave, and an intermittent low frequency wave with higher power. The whole process is commonly referred to as the "motility" of the GI tract.

Under usual circumstances, the rectum acts as a storage area for stool (sometimes known as doo-doo by us medical professionals). When the rectum is full, usually around 300 grams, a signal is sent by the nervous system to the brain that tells us to go to the bathroom and empty our bowels.

There is also a connection between the stomach and the rectum via the nervous system. When food distends the stomach, a message is relayed to the rectum that essentially says, "look out below", and causes an urge to defecate to make room for more. This is called the gastro-colic reflex.

Abnormalities in Irritable Bowel Syndrome

The pathology in IBS can basically be broken down into two categories: abnormalities in motility and dysfunctional sensation. Once again, the abnormalities vary from patient to patient so it has been difficult to explain the syndrome in terms of the individual. If we look at the disorder as stems from dysfunction in the control of bowel function by the central nervous system, the pathophysiology of IBS becomes much clearer.

Motility Problems

Some studies have shown an increase in slow-wave peristaltic contractions in the colon and rectum of patients with irritable bowel syndrome, but this finding has not been confirmed by all investigators (Snape, 1976). Diarrhea-predominant IBS patients have increased propulsion through the upper part of the colon, impairing the reabsorption of water and making the stool less solid (Vassallo, 1992). Small bowel contractility may also be hyperactive, which can lead to abdominal pain and distension (Kellow, 1987).

An abnormally sensitive gastro-colic reflex is a very common finding that has not been researched very well. The vast majority of IBS patients state that as soon as they eat or drink they have to run to the bathroom. This is not due to the popular notion that "everything runs right through me", but to an exaggerated gastro-colic reflex that occurs at smaller volumes of stool in the rectum. If the CNS tells you to empty your bowels with only 100 grams of stool, the bowel movement will be watery and unformed, another common characteristic of IBS.

Sensory Problems

The pain and bloating that often accompanies irritable bowel syndrome also occur because of an overly sensitive sensory system. Lasser and colleagues showed that the feelings of abdominal bloating and distension in IBS did not occur because of an increase in bowel gas, but rather that IBS patients experience symptoms at intestinal gas volumes that are lower than those that cause discomfort in normal subjects (Lasser, 1975).

Altered pain perception is common in IBS as well as in other types of Somatoneural Dysfunction. Several trials assessed pain threshold associated with distension of the rectum, small intestine, and sigmoid colon and found that IBS patients experienced symptoms at markedly smaller volumes than did normal control patients (Lynn, 1995). This altered visceral pain sensation has been shown to be a result of increased sensitivity of nerve endings along the GI tract and in the peripheral nerves that carry sensory information to the spinal cord (Mayer, 1990).

We also know that stress worsens IBS. This is due to neuroimmune mechanisms mediated primarily by cortisol and epinephrine release. This is actually a normal response seen in everyone (during my medical school final exams in my case) relating back to the fight-or-flight response. If you are being chased by a sabre-tooth tiger, you don't need to waste any time digesting your meal and achieving regular bowel movements, so energy is diverted away from the GI tract to the muscles and vascular system.

Other mechanisms contributing to abnormal pain perception in IBS have also been postulated. These include decreased levels of endorphins in cerebrospinal fluid, bile acid malabsorption in the small intestine, altered fluid secretion, and inflammation from local release of histamine from mast cells in the ileum. All of these theories have some supporting data, but no proven confirmatory studies.

Psychosocial Factors

In keeping with the tradition of other subtypes of Somatoneural Dysfunction, patients with irritable bowel syndrome have often been told their symptoms are entirely psychological by physicians who don't know any better. Psychiatric disorders such as depression, anxiety, and somatization disorder have been associated more frequently with patients who seek medical advice for IBS symptoms (Whitehead, 1988). However, those with IBS who did not seek medical attention had no higher rate of psychiatric pathology than those without IBS.

This leads to a conclusion that is central to the understanding of the manifestations of SND in general. Stress, anxiety, and depression often manifest as physical symptoms and most often cause the severity of the symptoms to increase. As we shall soon see, this is a two-way street. Affliction with an unknown set of symptoms (in this case diarrhea, constipation, or abdominal pain) can unmask or worsen symptoms of psychiatric distress.

Studies are conflicting with regards to the effect of stress on symptoms of IBS, but most patients experience an exacerbation of their symptoms when faced with acute or chronically stressful situations (Drossman, 1982). This is likely mediated through enhancement of the gastro-colic reflex as noted above as well as by direct nerve fibers from the brain connecting to the GI tract via the vagus nerve.

Relationship Between SND and IBS

Irritable bowel syndrome is a subtype of Somatoneural Dysfunction the same as fibromyalgia and chronic fatigue syndrome. Some patients have only symptoms of IBS, while others may have a combination of IBS symptoms with any of the other facets of SND. They all relate back to an abnormality in the way sensory information (in this case bowel function and abdominal distension) is interpreted by the central nervous system. Fortunately, IBS is manageable by using some of the same principles of treatment as other manifestations of SND as will be shown in Part 2.

Evaluation of Suspected Irritable Bowel Syndrome

Historically, the diagnosis of IBS is usually reached when all other possible causes of abdominal discomfort and altered bowel habits are excluded. This often necessitates a lengthy and expensive process that involves invasive procedures and subspecialist referrals. A more efficient diagnostic method is to use the clinical criteria noted above as a first step.

In many cases the diagnosis of IBS is quite clear from a simple history and physical examination. If the diagnosis is not clear, if existing symptoms worsen, or if new symptoms develop, it is imperative that further testing be done to clarify the situation and make sure another, potentially more severe, illness is not missed.

Typical evaluation if possible irritable bowel syndrome generally includes flexible sigmoidoscopy, stool analysis (for excess fat, ova and parasites, and white blood cells), and laboratory assessment (thyroid studies, erythrocyte sedimentation rate, complete blood count, and chemistry panel).

The presence of any of the following should elicit concern and prompt further investigation:

1. blood in the stool
2. fever or chills
3. weight loss
4. pain or diarrhea that interferes with sleep

Table 17: Diagnoses often Confuded With Irritable Bowel Syndrome

1. Colon cancer or villous adenoma
2. Inflammatory Bowel Disease (Crohn's Disease or ulcerative colitis)
3. Ischemic colitis (embolism or thrombosis of blood vessels)
4. Lactose intolerance (deficiency of the enzyme lactase)
5. Chronic idiopathic intestinal pseudo-obstruction
6. Parasitic infection (such as giardiasis)
7. Endometriosis
8. Depression, panic disorder, somatization disorder
9. Malabsorption syndromes (celiac sprue, Whipple's disease)
10. Pancreatic insufficiency
11. Fecal impaction
12. Medication side effects

Sick-Building Syndrome

Increases in energy-efficient buildings with recirculated air have led to the development of a specific type of Somatoneural Dysfunction that appears to be related to allergy and toxin sensitivity. Hallmark symptoms of sick-building syndrome (SBS) include upper respiratory irritation, headache, fatigue, and rash. Other symptoms common to SND may also occur along with irritative symptoms related to specific exposures (see below).

The clustering of cases necessitated investigation of infectious and toxic exposures, particularly in certain high-risk workplace environments such as nursing homes or industrial plants. Public awareness of epidemics of Legionnaire's disease and exposure to agents such as radon, asbestos, and secondary tobacco smoke have led to appropriate concern. It seems, however, that SBS is similar in manifestation to the old outbreaks of epidemic neuromyasthenia of the early investigation of chronic fatigue syndrome.

The study of sick-building syndrome overlaps with that of multiple chemical sensitivity. In fact, patients with both syndromes have neuro-psychiatric and allergic symptoms related to environmental exposures. The previous notion that these are two separate entities defies explanation, but illustrates how medical researchers have failed to notice the similarities among all types of Somatoneural Dysfunction for so long.

Table 18: Common Symptoms in Sick-Building Syndrome

Mucous-membrane Irritation	Respiratory	Skin	Chemosensory	Neurotoxic
Itchy, watery eyes	Cough	Rash	Visual changes	Headaches
Sore throat	Wheezing	Itchiness	Abnormal odors Fatigue	
Post-nasal drip	Dyspnea	Dryness	Dizziness	Poor concentration

These symptoms, though not severe or life threatening, can be quite annoying and unpleasant, causing lost productivity or work time and even disability. There can be obvious disruption to the work environment as several members of the workforce can be affected and fear of serious illness, communicable infection, or toxic exposure occurs.

Outbreaks seem to occur in the work environment as low-level exposure to substances with a toxic or allergic effect accumulates in susceptible patients. Environmental factors such as controlled humidity and temperature, poor indoor air quality, crowded office settings, and increased use of synthetic building components seem to be predisposing factors to SBS. Psychosocial factors such as stress, anxiety, and fatigue due to overwork seem to worsen the symptom complex.

In addition to this combination of factors, there appears to be a sensitivity to environmental factors in affected patients. There is some evidence for a heightened inflammatory response in these cases. Allergens and environmental toxins in a specific work environment trigger inflammatory and immune responses in SBS patients at lower levels of exposure than in others. Thus, this too is a subtype of Somatoneural Dysfunction and for all intents and purposes is indistinguishable from multiple chemical sensitivity.

Myofascial Pain Syndrome

Historically (by which I mean a few years ago, since most of what we know about these related disorders has been learned in the past few years), myofascial pain syndrome was distinct from fibromyalgia. It was defined as single or multiple trigger points throughout the body and often did not follow a characteristic pattern as seen in fibromyalgia. The latest definition of fibro really looks a lot like MPS with perhaps a stricter definition of the location of the trigger points.

It has also been stated that myofascial pain syndrome is a problem of the musculoskeletal system alone and not a system-wide disorder as in the other types of Somatoneural Dysfunction. I myself believe that MPS is a symptom of SND and not a true disorder itself. There is a spectrum of myofascial trigger/tender points in people that range from normal (everyone has a few at certain times in their lives) to pathologic (multiple, widespread, severe).

We do, however, need to understand the concept of the myofascial trigger point in the context of Somatoneural Dysfunction. Myofascia is a tough, fibrous connective tissue that covers muscle tissue and helps to supply muscles with nutrients, blood flow, protection, and strengthening. It also is present in specific strengthening and connecting structures like tendons and ligaments. Fascia is an embryologic tissue that exists as a three-dimensional web covering the body from head to foot. It organizes along lines of tension in the body and contracts to protect against trauma while adding support to prevent misalignment.

Myofascia is classified into three categories:
1. Superficial: lying directly below the dermis
2. Deep: surrounding organs, muscle, bone, nerves, and blood vessels
3. Deepest: encasing the central nervous system and the brain (Ramsay, 1997).

The connective tissue is comprised of three main components: collagen, elastin, and ground substance. Collagen is a protein that is made up of polypeptide chains that act like a cable and provides much of the strength to the tissue. Elastin adds, oddly enough, elasticity necessary for stretch and recoil of tendons and arteries. Ground substance is a gelatinous polysaccharide complex that helps absorb compressive forces and distribute mechanical shock and strain (Guyton, 2000).

When myofascia loses some of its elasticity and strength it can become knotted, weakened, and taut. Over time, this fascial strain can tighten and act to pull the body out of alignment, causing inefficient movement and posture. Bundles of adhesions or scar tissue can form and lead to the occurrence of tender points when stretched or pressed. Pain may also be "referred" when the trigger point is irritated, sending pain along the length of the myofascial connections.

Trigger points and myofascial pain syndrome have been thought to sometimes lead to weakness in the related muscle groups, but this is probably not true.

Table 19: Clinical Characteristics of Myofascial Pain Syndrome	
Trigger Points in Taut Band of Muscle - tenderness on palpation - consistent points of tenderness - palpation alters pain - alleviation with extinction of trigger points	Referred Pain - constant dull ache - fluctuates in intensity - consistent pattern of referral
Contributing Factors - paresthesias - gastrointestinal upset - visual disturbances - dermatographia - hearing disturbances	Associated Symptoms - trauma/whiplash - repetitive strain injury - sleep disturbance - disuse atrophy - psychosocial/emotional stress (Fricton, 1997)

Studies done in fibromyalgia patients showed that maximal power and strength of muscle groups was about the same as normal patients, but maximal exertion was accompanied by more pain during the activity and more exhaustive symptoms afterwards. A

Some authors make a distinction between trigger points and tender points. Tender points hurt where touched, while trigger points hurt in a distribution along adjacent nerve roots. Pathologically, I think they are the same, except that trigger points occur near nerve bundles that refer pain.

trigger point is typically a 2-5 mm point of hypersensitivity located in knotted bands of muscle, tendon, or ligament. These points may be active or latent: active points are continuously painful, while latent points are only painful when palpated. The pattern of pain is altered by palpation, either increased or decreased, and is consistently reproducible. Often, patients will withdraw or jump when the trigger point is pressed. Referred pain from trigger points is along specific lines of myofascia. Generally, local treatments at the trigger point will relieve the referred pain if pain is relieved at the trigger point.

Associated muscle groups may be easily fatigued and stiff. They may be painful when moved or stretched, resulting in compensatory abnormalities in posture or activity that actually worsen the overall pain. There may be a sense of weakness or restriction in range of motion, but this is almost always due to an attempt to lessen pain that true decreased strength of the involved muscle groups.

Accompanying sensory abnormalities are common. Paresthesias, such as tingling or numbness along the line of referred pain, occur in about 30% of patients, particularly if the trigger points are close to superficial nerve branches. Visual disturbances may include excessive tearing, blurred vision, and twitching or trembling of the eyes, while ringing in the ears, decreased hearing, dizziness, ear pain can also be seen. It is unclear why these symptoms occur in conjunction with myofascial pain, but is probably due to myofascial abnormalities in the intrinsic muscles and connective tissue of the eyes and inner ears.

Stress can make myofascial trigger points worse. Hans Selye, one of the most brilliant physiologist and behaviorists of this century, believed that a process of calcification occurred in myofascia in response to stress (Starlanyl, 1996). However, more recent studies have concluded that this is probably not true. Stress probably worsens trigger point tenderness in the same manner it worsens Somatoneural Dysfunction in general, by suppressing immune system and HPAA function and leading to a state of neurologic hyperirritability.

Maladaptive behaviors tend to worsen the trigger points and overall disability from myofascial pain and SND. This includes poor posture, lack of exercise leading to disuse and muscle atrophy, poor sleep and dietary habits, medication dependency, anxiety, depression, and frustration. Muscle tension-producing habits, such as back bracing, neck tensing, and teeth clenching may also worsen the problem.

The pathology underlying myofascial pain and trigger points remains to be fully elicited. Under the microscope, affected muscle and connective tissue do not reveal signs of inflammation as originally suspected. Instead they show abnormalities in mitochondria, the energy source of cells. Some have also seen infiltration of fat cells, fibrocytes, or lymphocytes, but these results have been inconsistent.

The decrease in muscle energy (ATP) seen in muscle biopsy specimens suggests lack of oxygen in tissues associated with trigger points. This also leads to an increase in toxic products of muscle metabolism such as lactate, which leads to increased fatigue in the affected muscle groups. Inflammatory mediators may be released, further contributing to pain, and calcium deposits can build up on associated ligaments and tendons and within local joint spaces.

This cascade of events can be initiated by traumatic events (either acute or repetitive) or by sustained muscular tension and may continue to worsen even after the initial stimulus has resolved. This in turn creates muscle hypersensitivity and leads to decay of the connective fibers, which results in the formation of myofascial bundles.

As with other similar syndromes, mechanical factors and psychiatric aspects of illness play a role in worsening the symptom complex. The pain decreases ability to exercise, which leads to deconditioning. Learned avoidance behavior further complicates the issue and makes it even less likely that a patient will be able to break this vicious cycle on their own.

Figure 5: Formation of Trigger Points

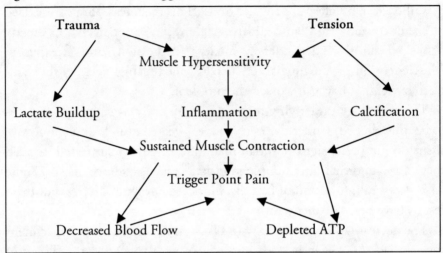

It is therefore easy to see why this type of painful process is so hard to treat on occasion. We may be able to temporarily interrupt the process by disrupting the ascending pain pathways with local treatment or pain relievers, or by modulating the central pain response. The cycle, however, needs to be broken at some point to prevent ongoing damage and pain. Only then can each contributing factor be assessed and corrected by a multidisciplinary approach designed to:

1) restore local blood flow
2) decrease inflammation
3) restore muscle energy in the form of ATP
4) lessen sustained muscle contraction.

Gulf War Syndrome

The newest entry in the subtypes of Somatoneural Dysfunction has been termed Gulf War Syndrome, to describe a characteristic set of symptoms experienced by many combat veterans returning home from the Persian Gulf after the 1991 conflict. Several theories tried to relate the syndrome to infectious or environmental exposures or attribute the symptoms to post-traumatic stress disorder. This follows a pattern that should be all too familiar at this point in the book.

Symptoms of Gulf War Syndrome serve as a nice illustration of the overall effect of Somatoneural Dysfunction. If we use previously mentioned criteria for diagnosis of other related subtypes of SND, about 30% fit into the category of chronic fatigue syndrome, another 25% seem to have fibromyalgia, and an additional 10% match the symptoms of multiple chemical hypersensitivity. This approximates the distribution of Somatoneural Dysfunction in general, with a slightly increased predominance of CFS. The remainder of the patients have an overlap of symptoms from two or more categories (Pollet, 1998).

An editorial in 1997 printed in the Journal of the American Medical Association acknowledged this link:

> "Physicians need to acknowledge that many Gulf War veterans
> are experiencing stress-related disorders and the physical
> consequences of stress. These conditions should not be hidden
> or denied, but rather are well-recognized entities that have been
> studied extensively in survivors of past wars, most notably the
> Vietnam conflict. As physicians, we should not accept a
> diagnosis of stress-related disorders in veterans prior to exclud
> physical factors, but at the same time, we need to recognize the
> pervasive presence of stress-related illness such as hypertension,
> fibromyalgia, and chronic fatigue among Persian Gulf War
> veterans and manage these illnesses appropriately. As a nation
> we must get beyond the fallacious idea that diseases of the
> mind are either not real or are shameful and to better
> recognize that the mind and the body are inexorably linked"
> (Ismail, 1999)

This could be the theme to the book you are now reading if not for the lack of reference to the very real biological dysfunction present in SND and Gulf War syndrome.

Symptoms of diffuse aches and pain, upper respiratory problems (wheezing, itchy eyes, runny nose, and cough), and profound fatigue are most common. When compared to control groups of veterans deployed in non-combat positions in Germany during the Gulf War, Persian-deployed veterans experienced a wide variety of non-specific symptoms:

- neurological (dizziness, numbness, referred pain, headaches)
- gastrointestinal (diarrhea, abdominal bloating, cramping)
- cardiac (palpitations, tachycardia)
- dermatologic (itching, temperature change in skin)
- musculoskeletal (joint pain, weakness, muscle spasm)
- neuropsychiatric (poor memory, lack of concentration, depression)

The subjects variously thought their symptoms were due to debris from SCUD missile attacks, exposure to pesticides, use of biological or chemical weapons, anticholinesterase agents used as a precaution against chemical weapon attacks, or smoke from tent heaters (Proctor, 1998). Attempts to correlate symptoms with any of these exposures have been unsuccessful.

More recent studies have found a similar spectrum of symptoms in British veterans of the Bosnian conflict, making it unlikely that chemical weapon exposure or environmental factors could be responsible for the syndrome (Ismail, 1999).

So, if it is not caused by environmental or chemical exposures, what is the cause? I suspect it is the same as the cause for Somatoneural Dysfunction, an oversensitive connection between the central nervous system and other related organ systems amplified by significant stress and psychological factors. Lack of quality sleep probably also worsens the clinical symptoms of the syndrome.

Investigation of the musculoskeletal pain that often accompanies Gulf War syndrome fails to show any evidence of inflammatory or rheumatic condition (Escalante, 1998). Some patients have myofascial trigger points while others were found to have only some minimal evidence of osteoarthritis or arthralgias. Profiles of allergy and immune system abnormalities have shown no differences between veterans and control populations, although veterans with allergies definitely experienced significantly worse upper respiratory symptoms than those without (Klaustmayer, 1998).

Anxiety and stress worsen existing symptoms of pain and fatigue in Gulf War syndrome the same way they do in fibromyalgia. This syndrome should provide a lot of information on the pathogenesis of Somatoneural Dysfunction if the medical field can overcome our tendency to try and attribute it to an infection or environmental toxin.

It is very likely that decreased levels of serotonin in the brain and increased substance P in nerve terminals combined with subtle immune and endocrine dysregulation are also responsible for Gulf War syndrome. Already, some studies have begun to investigate how wartime stress alters cytokine and lymphocyte function (Everson, 1999), while others are looking at the physical manifestations of Post-Traumatic Stress Disorder.

In the battle against Somatoneural Dysfunction, Gulf War Syndrome has presented researchers with a well-defined population sample to study. We were able to see clearly how previously healthy, physically fit, and mentally well-trained young men and women responded to acute, persistent stressors that accompany armed conflict. They developed fibromyalgia, irritable bowel syndrome, multiple chemical sensitivity, and chronic fatigue syndrome.

With all this evidence from observational and epidemiological study, it is mind-boggling that efforts continue to be squandered on eliciting an infectious or environmental cause. The good news thus far is that most veterans afflicted with Gulf War illness have an excellent capacity for recovery with a treatment program consisting of physical and cognitive therapy along with specific medical regimens designed to alleviate symptoms, just like others with Somatoneural Dysfunction.

Some experts have concluded that Gulf War Syndrome must be a neurologic condition, much in the same way that I have explained SND as a neuorologic condition in these pages. Soon, I hope we will come full circle and realize the connectivity between all these ailments. Only then can we truly begin to understand the nature of the illness and fully begin to make patients better.

Chapter 5:
Psychiatric Aspects of Somatoneural Dysfunction

A very useful book about understanding and coping with Somatoneural Dysfunction, entitled "Fibromyalgia and Chronic Myofascial Pain Syndrome: A Survival Manual" is written by Dr. Devin Starlanyl and Mary Ellen Copeland, two sufferers of these syndromes and noted authors in the field. I highly recommend the book for patients as a simple, easy to read guide for coping. However, there are several flaws in the book, the most prominent being that there is virtually no mention of the impact of psychiatric factors on the syndrome. I find it a bit odd that these authors, Ms. Copeland (author of several fine works on living with depression, from which she also suffers) in particular, fail to acknowledge and discuss the link between SND and psychiatric disorders such as depression (Starlanyl, 1996).

This illustrates a point that, even today as 24 million Americans suffer from Major Depression and millions more from minor depression (dysthymia), people are loath to admit it. Part of the reason why advocates for fibromyalgia and other SND subtypes avoid discussion of how depression relates to their disorder is due to the persisting stigma of mental illness. These patients are particularly sensitive to this negative labeling because it is likely that they have been told for years that their medical condition was "all in your head".

Unfortunately, now that a physiological basis for the symptoms of Somatoneural Dysfunction has been identified, there is a shift in the opposite direction to claim that SND has nothing to due with psychiatric factors. This goes too far in the other direction. In order to maximize understanding and effective treatments for SND, one has to realize and accept the way the physiology interacts with the psychology. We know from chapter 2 that stress and other psychological factors impact directly on biologic function, so this observation should come as no surprise.

Starlanyl and Copeland state that the prevalence of psychiatric disorders in fibromyalgia is "no higher than in other chronic pain syndromes". This fact may be true, but the rate of coexisting depression in fibromyalgia and related syndromes, as well as other chronic pain syndromes may be as high as 70%. Certainly, a percentage this high is nothing to be overlooked.

Unfortunately, an inherent bias is almost always present when the physician is treating patients with the same illness as the doctor. There is too often a striking sense that "because this works for me, it will work for you too". A reliance on personal anecdotal evidence, rather than controlled clinical data is the other serious flaw in Dr. Starlanyl's work. She all too frequently sites things like, "Three patients experienced improvement in hardness from their breast implants while on guaifenesin therapy". Observational data does play an incredibly significant role in formulating medical research, but to base therapy recommendations on uncontrolled findings involving 3 patients may be a bit irresponsible.

One reason for depressive manifestations in Somatoneural Dysfunction is painfully clear (no pun intended of course). If you don't feel good all day, suffer from terrible aches and pains, sleep poorly, and are unable to function to your best ability all day, you may become depressed. It is only common sense. There are certainly patients with SND who are not depressed and depressed patients without SND, but the overlap is considerable. Alternatively, we also know that depressive illnesses are commonly manifested by the perception of physical illness. Depression can act as a great magnifier of pain, fatigue, and a variety of other symptoms. Added to the already hypersensitive neural networks in SND and you can easily see why the potential amplification of physical symptoms is such an important problem in patients with coexisting major depressive disorder.

The reciprocal relationship between SND and depression makes it imperative that depressive symptoms are identified and treated as part of a multimodal treatment program. In my experience, failure to identify and treat depression in SND is one of the primary reasons for treatment failure. This is due to a combination of physician reluctance to seek out "psychiatric" disorders and patients' wish to avoid being labeled as such.

Ok, So What is Depression?

Depression is a disorder of mood that occurs as a result from a combination of environmental, genetic, and biochemical factors. Dysthymia, or minor depression (a name I do not particularly care for) is similar in nature, but lessened somewhat in severity. The criteria for each are listed in the following tables and are according to the Diagnostic and Statistic Manual-IV (DSM-IV), which is the standard of the American Psychiatric Association.

Despite the fact that depression affects nearly one of every five people at some point during their lifetime, physicians are still woefully inept at diagnosing and treating it correctly. In a 1990 study, primary care providers made an accurate diagnosis of depression in only 35.7% of patients (Perez-Stable, 1990). The cost to society of lost productivity due to non-treatment of depression spirals into billions.

In patients with medical illness, the incidence of depression increases up to 57% or more, and generally follows the common sense caveat that the sicker a patient is, the more likely they are to be depressed (Katon,

1990). Unfortunately, many patients (and physicians) believe that this type of depression is not treatable. In fact, treating depression with psychotherapy and/or medication therapy improves quality of life, relieves depressive symptoms, and possibly even improves the medical problem as well. A landmark study done in Britain showed that survival from metastatic breast cancer was increased by group psychotherapy. The therapy group survived an amazing 36.6 months compared to the standard treatment group's survival rate of 18.9 months, nearly twice as long (Spiegel, 1989). If this doesn't hit home the importance of the mind in treating medical illness, nothing will.

Therefore, a search for signs of depression in Somatoneural Dysfunction certainly seems reasonable, as the two disorders share many physiologic and psychologic parameters. There are several diagnostic questionnaires designed to help determine whether or not a patient is depressed. Beck's and Hamilton's Depression Inventory are two of the most commonly used. More recently, the PRIME-MD has become popular.

Table 20: DSM-IV Criteria for Major Depressive Episode

Five or more of the following symptoms have been present during the same 2-week period and represents a change from previous level of functioning; at least one of either 1) depressed mood or 2) loss of interest or pleasure must be present

1) depressed mood most of the day, nearly every day (can be observed by others, or expressed by the patient)
2) markedly diminished interest or pleasure in all, or almost all, activities most of the day, nearly every day (as observed or expressed)
3) weight loss or gain of more than 5% of body weight in a one month period, or increase or decrease in appetite nearly every day.

---

4) Insomnia or hypersomnia nearly every day
5) Observed psychomotor agitation or slowing nearly every day
6) Fatigue or loss of energy nearly every day
7) Feelings of worthlessness or excessive or inappropriate guilt nearly every day
8) Diminished ability to think or concentrate, or indecisiveness nearly every day
9) Recurrent thoughts of death or a suicide attempt

The symptoms cause clinically significant distress or impairment in social, occupational, or other important areas of functioning.

If you have Somatoneural Dysfunction, these symptoms will likely sound remarkably familiar once again. Strictly speaking, major depressive disorder is exclusive of symptoms related to a medical condition. However, depression in Somatoneural Dysfunction can happen as an indirect result of the chronic, incapacitating symptoms of the disorder. Actually, this kind of "secondary depression" can be seen with any severe medical illness.

Certainly, a lack of interest in doing activities for pleasure (anhedonia) is common in SND. I ask my patients a simple question: "What do you do for fun?" A typical response will be "Nothing!" The day is usually consumed with the effort it takes to go to work or school and to care for one's family, leaving become available specifically designed for primary care physicians to use as a quick and efficient screening tool. This 26-question, self-administered instrument proved to be 98% specific at diagnosing depression. This means that if the PRIME-MD indicates that depression is present, 98% of the time the diagnosis is confirmed on more comprehensive testing. It must be kept in mind that the test is not very sensitive (i.e. good at ruling out depression) as depression or depressive symptoms may still be present in many of the patients who have a negative PRIME-MD (Spitzer, 1994). If major depressive disorder is still suspected, referral to a psychiatrist is necessary for a more thorough evaluation. Depressed mood is also quite common, usually stemming from despair over the symptoms of SND, anger and resentment at being unable to find an answer or a treatment, and fears of serious medical and emotional illness. Irritability of mood can be as much an indication of depression as depressed mood.

Insomnia or hypersomnia can be part of the spectrum of sleep pathology present in Somatoneural Dysfunction. Sleep disturbances are very common in depressive disorders and may include abnormal slow-wave sleep, delayed sleep onset, and dysfunctional REM sleep. Fatigue and loss of energy are most prominent in chronic fatigue syndrome, but are also common in other subtypes as well. Similarly, lack of concentration or memory deficits is frequently present. If you have those five criteria, you will most likely fit the diagnosis of major depression.

The other symptoms listed in the criteria for major depression, though less common, may also be present in SND at various times and be of variable severity. It then seems to be reasonable to conclude that depression at least shares a lot in common with Somatoneural Dysfunction. It appears that SND patients are particularly susceptible to depression at times when their illness flares.

Dysthmia is a more chronic, but less severe counterpart to major depression. It is very common, affecting up to 5% of people in this country at any given time. Combined with the 10-25% of Americans who experience depression at one time or another, one has to wonder why there is such a negative stigma on such a common problem. Depression and dysthymia

Table 21: Dysthymia in DSM-IV
A. Depressed mood for most of the day, for more days than not (observed or expressed)
B. Two or more of the following
•   Poor appetite or overeating
•   Insomnia or hypersomnia
•   Low energy or fatigue
•   Low self-esteem
•   Poor concentration or indecisiveness
•   Feelings of hopelessness

appear to share many common physiological features with Somatoneural Dysfunction.

Neuroendocrine abnormalities are common to major depressive disorder and Somatoneural Dysfunction and can include a blunted response to stimulation of cortisol, thyroid hormone, and growth hormone release (Kaplan and Sadock, 1998). Dysregulation of the immune response and alterations of blood flow to certain areas of the brain in depression are also similar in nature to those seen in SND.

Perhaps the most consistent and striking finding in depression is the abnormality in the serotonin system. Levels of serotonin are low in the cerebrospinal fluid (CSF) of depressed patients. Furthermore, there are decreased numbers of serotonin receptors on certain cells. Experimental reduction in the level of serotonin has lead to depressive symptoms in research settings.

I like to think of serotonin as the brain's "missile defense system" against invasion by depressive thoughts and symptoms. Each time something depressing happens, the serotonin system fires a volley of missiles to effectively neutralize the threat. You get divorced, a missile fires. You lose your job, a missile fires. You get involved in a car accident, another missile fires. Your mother-in-law comes to stay with you for a month, six missiles fire. Sometimes the missile defense system is overwhelmed or depleted. No more serotonin-laden missiles are available, and depression occurs. I believe this is an important part of Somatoneural Dysfunction as well, whether this is an inciting event or a resultant effect remains to be seen.

The norepinephrine and dopamine systems are also involved in depression and SND. Norepinephrine works on the sympathetic nervous system by its action on β-receptors, which are present in blood vessels, nerve endings, and smooth muscle. These receptors are also located on neurons of the serotonin system and play a role in regulating the release of serotonin. The D1-type of dopamine receptor is reduced in number and function and may be defective in SND as well.

More on the Relationship Between SND and Depression, Please

Depression may precede symptoms of SND or patients with SND may become depressed. Medical theorists have debated the point of which one causes the other until they are blue in their collective faces. For me, however, it is only of academic interest. More important is that depression is a frequent and important part of Somatoneural Dysfunction and must always be assessed and treated if present. To ignore this is to do a grave disservice to patients and miss a potentially treatable diagnosis that can be lethal if missed.

There are three basic theories of the relationship between Somatoneural Dysfunction and depression:

1) SND may be a manifestation of depression. However, the majority of patients were not depressed at the time their symptoms developed. The response of many patients with SND to antidepressant medications favored this theory, but the typical dose of medication needed is much lower than that in depression and probably signifies the overlap in neuro-transmitter abnormality seen in both conditions.

2) Depression may be a manifestation of SND. This certainly makes sense, as virtually all disorders that have chronic pain and malaise have high rates of coexisting depression. The longer a patient suffers with SND without appropriate treatment, the more likely they are to become depressed.

3) A common basic trait is shared by SND and depression. This theory includes depression and syndromes such as fibromyalgia and chronic fatigue syndrome into "affective spectrum disorders" by pointing out the many common-alities between them. Many researchers resist this, as they do the classification of Somatoneural Dysfunction, on epidemiological grounds that it hinders research (Goldenberg, 1989). I would argue

that by lumping these disorders together, we will gain further insight into their pathogenesis and treatment; a much more important goal to clinicians and patients.

Fibromyalgia is probably the most studied type of SND in regards to depressive symptoms. Interestingly, if you read most of the books on the shelf next to this one in a bookstore, they fail to acknowledge the link between fibromyalgia and depression. Many early research studies compared the prevalence of depression in fibromyalgia to rheumatoid arthritis. Those studies that showed that differences were generally too small in number to detect such a trend. The largest, by Hawley and Wolfe in 1993, looked at over 1500 patients with either fibromyalgia or RA. The FM patients showed a significant increase in depressive symptoms (Hawley, 1993). Another randomized trial done in 1991 found an increase in depression among FM patients, but the difference was not large (Ahles, 1991). Virtually every study of fibromyalgia has shown a major increase in depressive symptoms as compared to patients without fibromyalgia. Preliminary results in other chronic fatigue syndromes appear similar.

I believe this data is best explained in terms of Somatoneural Dysfunction as follows:
1. Clinical depression is common in SND
2. Not all SND patients are depressed
3. All patients with SND should be screened for depression
4. Depression makes the symptoms of SND worse
5. Depression is a treatable part of SND

Figure 6: Classical Theory of Affective Spectrum Disorders

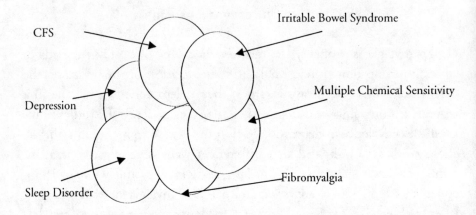

In this view, there is an overlap in the clinical and pathologic factors of depression and many of the subtypes of Somatoneural Dysfunction. Despite this intricate association, the syndromes have historically all been viewed as distinct entities. The failure to unite all of these disorders under a single, comprehensive syndrome has been one of the major obstacles to effective research and design of treatment programs that addresses the whole spectrum of symptoms. Another problem inherent in this model, of course, is that no one has been quite certain how they all fit together. Often, researchers will isolate one syndrome in order to study it and exclude the presence of others. For example, in many early studies of fibromyalgia and chronic fatigue syndrome, researchers did not include any patient with depression. Now, as we have said, there is up to a 70% rate of patients with FMS/CFS who have features of major depression. It seems to me that a patient with chronic pain and fatigue without depressive features is an uncommon finding and may represent a whole different spectrum of disease manifestation. These early studies were important in allowing us to determine that fibromyalgia (for example) is a distinct entity from major depression, but that they nevertheless share many common features.

I prefer to describe an overlap between SND and depression that encompasses each individual syndrome. This allows a better understanding of the true relationship to one another. Depression may touch upon each individual syndrome as an integral part of SND, be related independently to SND, or stand alone without physical manifestations.

Figure 7: My Theory of Somatoneural Dysfunction

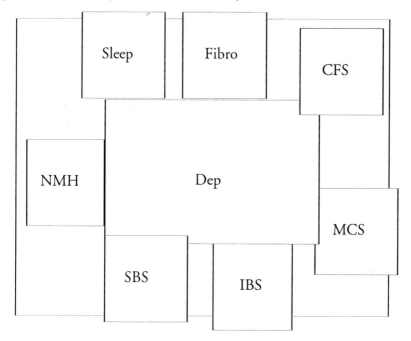

Key to abbreviations: CFS: chronic fatigue syndrome
Fibro: fibromyalgia
MCS: multiple chemical sensitivity
SBS: sick building syndrome
IBS: irritable bowel syndrome

Sleep: sleep disorders
Dep: secondary depression
NMH: neurally-mediated hypotension
SND: Somatoneural Dysfunction

Other Psychiatric Factors

Panic Attacks

It is quite common for patients with Somatoneural Dysfunction to suffer from panic attacks. These episodes are char-acterized by a feeling of impending doom, often accompanied by rapid or irregular pulse rate, rapid breathing, pains in the chest, throat tight-ness, dizziness or light-headedness, or nausea and stomach upset. People who experience these attacks often find their way to emergency rooms and become themselves victims of un-necessary and inva-sive testing.

The study by Ahles and associates looked at panic disorder in fibro-myalgia and showed an incidence

Table 22: Panic Disorder (DSM-IV)
A discrete period of fear or discomfort which develops suddenly and peaks within ten minutes. Four or more of the following must be present.
1) palpitations, rapid or pounding heart
2) sweating
3) trembling or shaking
4) sensation of shortness of breath or smothering
5) feeling of choking
6) chest pain or discomfort
7) nausea or abdominal distress
8) feeling dizzy, lightheaded, unsteady, or faint
9) derealization or depersonalization (feelings of detachment or unreality)
10) fear of losing control or going crazy
11) fear of dying
12) numbness or tingling sensations
13) chills or hot flushes

nearly five times that of control patients and more than twice that of those with rheumatoid arthritis. Panic disorder is characterized by recurrent attacks accompanied by more than a month of fear of having the attacks or the con-sequences (i.e. going crazy, losing control, having a heart attack) of the attacks. This fear results in a significant change in behavior. Panic attacks that occur in response to a specific stimulus (heights, crowds, spiders, etc) are called phobias.

A panic attack is really just a manifestation of an overactive sympathetic nervous system. This system, often called the "fight-or-flight" response, is designed to protect us and get us out of danger. It does this by releasing epinephrine and norepinephrine, which then act to speed up the heart and respiratory rates and cause the heart to beat more forcefully in order to supply the muscles with enough blood to fight or run away. This diverts nutrients and blood supply away from the other systems and can result in malfunction. This sensation of cardiovascular or pulmonary distress triggers other symptoms (listed in Table 17) of the fear and avoidance response.

This emergency response system is quite useful when you're being chased once again by a sabre-tooth tiger, but can be quite an inconvenience on a crowded subway car. For some patients, a specific situation triggers a panic attack, especially being chased by a sabre-tooth tiger. Many times, however, the inciting event may not even be noticed by the patient. A fleeting thought, possibly initiated by something seen out of the corner of the eye, a smell, or a sound, may trigger the attack. Physical symptoms, such as pain, upper respiratory problems, dizziness, or stomach upset are notorious for triggering attacks. These symptoms can all be due to perfectly benign conditions but can cause such anxiety and upset that an attack may be incited.

In SND, the sympathetic nervous system is quite sensitive to such triggers. This is likely also due to low levels of serotonin and dysregulation of serotonin receptor sensitivity. An imbalance between the serotonin and norepinephrine system may exist, or the norepinephrine system may be hypersensitive itself.

Somatoform Disorders

According to the American Psychiatric Association, the somatoform disorders are characterized by physical symptoms that have no basis in medical findings and cause significant distress and impaired functioning. I believe that many, if not most, of the patients formerly classified in this category actually have Somatoneural Dysfunction.

The DSM-IV describes five subtypes of somatoform disorder:

1) Somatization disorder: a combination of pain, gastro-intestinal distress, sexual dysfunction, and neurologic symptoms.
2) Conversion disorder: predominantly neurologic symptoms that usually occur after some type of traumatic event.
3) Hypochondriasis: preoccupation with the belief that a "normal" bodily function is indicative of a serious disease.
4) Pain disorder: intractable symptoms without physical evidence.
5) Body dysmorphic disorder: belief that a part of one's body is abnormal.

I am suspicious that, at least in the first four subtypes of somatoform disorder, Somatoneural Dysfunction plays a primary role in the pathogenesis of these symptoms. It's possible that the medical profession has overlooked the subtle, but real physiological abnormalities of SND and labeled these patients with a purely psychiatric disorder. Certainly, as I have described, psychiatric factors play an integral role in the onset and course of Somatoneural Dysfunction, but it would be an extremely rare case that is purely psychological. Therefore, in some cases I would favor the elimination of this classification from certain patients and would include them as a subtype of SND.

Diagnosis of somatization disorder relies on the presence of symptoms of diffuse pain (as may be seen in any myofascial pain syndrome), gastrointestinal upset (irritable bowel would fit in here quite nicely), sexual dysfunction (which is a common manifestation of concomitant depression in SND), and neurological signs (such as parasthesias or weakness) whose true pathology could be easily overlooked.

Other symptoms of Somatoneural Dysfunction could be misdiagnosed as a mild case of conversion disorder. Abnormalities in sensation or movement may fall into this category, although more severe symptoms like psychogenic blindness, seizures, or ataxia are less likely to be misinterpreted.

Hypochondriac in the traditional "Felix Unger" sense implies a person that sees every physical symptom as a harbinger of a serious medical illness. This may be similar in nature to the amplification of symptom severity that occurs due to dysfunctional transfer of sensory input into the central nervous system in SND. Given the elusive nature of the cause of Somatoneural Dysfunction and the lack of knowledge by the medical profession, it's quite possible that patients with SND could be diagnosed with hypochondriasis. Hypochondriasis may simply be another aspect of SND where the symptoms vary over time and have a broad range of manifestations.

Pain Disorder, for all intents and purposes, could be applied to any patient with fibromyalgia if the diagnosis of FM was not reached. Its diagnosis is made by simply having multiple areas of pain that cause significant distress or impairment of social functionality. Certainly, before we knew what fibromyalgia was, all of these patients could be lumped into this category.

Interestingly, treatment recommendations for most patients classified as having somatoform disorder includes medications that raise levels of serotonin, physical therapy, and cognitive-behavioral therapy. This follows much the same pathway for treatment of other types of SND.

The Sick Role

The belief that one is sick can be a powerful one and may contribute heavily to the severity of Somatoneural Dysfunction symptoms. This phenomenon is not, however, unique to SND, but plays a role in virtually all disease processes. An intriguing study done in the late 1970s assessed how the knowledge of one's illness affected its impact on a patient's life. Patients missed three times more work once they were diagnosed and treated for hypertension. This effect was independent of the treatment regimen (Haynes, 1978). Patients whose hypertension was mild and required no specific medical treatment still missed much more work than those with mild hypertension who were not told.

Other studies have looked at the beliefs of patients about their illness and how it affects illness duration and severity. Patients who believed themselves to have a poor immune system or to have a hard time fighting off colds had more severe and enduring symptoms than those who believed themselves better able to fight off infections (Cope, 1994). Dozens of other studies in ailments as diverse as heart disease, herpes zoster, and lactose intolerance have proven that patient belief about the severity of their illness can predict outcome (Barsky, 1999). This is an amazing finding that has largely been overlooked in the medical field, despite having tremendous potential as part of a therapeutic program for a multitude of disease states. The treatment chapters in Part 2 will delve into this more fully.

Suggestion can amplify and maintain symptoms. Doctors and patients have known for centuries (with and without benefit of formal controlled studies) that positive thinking and coping strategies can be beneficial in the course of illness. Similarly, negative beliefs and poor coping strategies often lead to adverse effects.

A large, multicenter study of aspirin in the treatment of heart disease also assessed the rate of gastrointestinal side effects. Patients who were told that aspirin may lead to stomach upset were six times more likely to report such effects than those who were not told (Myers, 1987). In my practice, I tell patients that every medicine can cause every side effect, and do not mention specifics unless there is a very specific, severe effect that is related to a certain medicine I am prescribing. Rather, I encourage patients to report to me any unusual symptom they experience while on a new medication. This seems to work out fine, and may be the safest way to assess medication side effects. I have not, however, been able to determine for one of my patients if the erythromycin I gave her for bronchitis was what caused all of her parrot's feathers to fall off...

A study was done, rather cruelly I think, to determine whether the power of suggestion could be used to produce headaches. Volunteers were told that a mild electrical current was going to be passed through their heads and asked to tell whether they got headaches or not. No real electrical current was used, but the vast majority of subjects reported headache symptoms anyway (Schweiger, 1981)

These studies illustrate how powerful beliefs can be in contributing to illness severity and duration. This can be combated, at least partially, simply by explanation. By adjusting expectations and beliefs of patients to a more beneficial (and hopefully accurate) assessment of the disease state, potential ill effects of negative beliefs can be overcome. My patients with Somatoneural Dysfunction commonly come into my office not knowing why they feel so poorly, and half expecting to die within the next six months from some dreaded, unknown disease. If I am able to explain what they are experiencing and why, in a manner that they can understand, we are on the first step to recovery together.

If I can't, or a patient is unfortunate enough to have a medical team without experience in dealing with SND, the patient may enter into the "sick role". The theory holds that once a patient is labeled as ill, they are regarded and treated differently by doctors, family, and society. Recovery is often hindered as continued illness may become expected of the patient.

In today's health care climate, the sick role can be complicated by the effect of disability payments, litigation, and worker's compensation.

Patients are often forced to prove that they are ill to receive justifiable benefits. This is part of the reason why patients with disability claims often have poorer outcomes for similar problems that those without claims (work-related versus non-work related carpal tunnel syndrome). Both the medical and legal professions have had difficulty interpreting this process and unfortunately, the overall effect on a patient's health may be misconstrued as malingering.

Post-Traumatic Stress Disorder

In 1871, DaCosta described symptoms of neurologic hyperarousal, psychologic numbness, rapid heart rate and breathing, chest tightness, and palpitations that came on in intermittent waves. He was studying young, healthy combat soldiers without any evidence of organic heart disease and labeled the syndrome "Irritable Heart". His classic findings over a century ago were probably closer to the truth than many researchers who came much later. Now we know that the "irritability" stems from the sympathetic nervous system and causes an effect on the heart and many other organ systems.

During World War I, this same syndrome was called "shell shock", while it was known as combat neurosis or operational fatigue in World War II. The term "posttraumatic stress disorder" (PTSD) was coined during the Vietnam War when it was realized that increasing severity of stress made it more likely for the syndrome to develop. About 30% of Vietnam veterans experience some degrees of symptoms from PTSD, but it is by no means limited only to soldiers. Some estimates state that PTSD may affect up to 3% of people at some point in their lives.

Biological factors that appear to contribute to the onset of posttraumatic stress disorder are nearly identical to those seen with other types of Somatoneural Dysfunction and include:

- Hyperactivity of the noradrenergic part of the sympathetic nervous system

- Dysfunction of endogenous opioid receptors
- Hypersensitive hypothalamic-pituitary-adrenal axis
- Sleep fragmentation and delayed onset
- Coexisting depression, anxiety, and panic disorder

A common psychological feature is alexithymia. This is an inability to identify or express inner feelings, which may lead to manifestation of physical symptoms. Sigmund Freud was the champion of this theory and it may still apply to patients with SND today. This is one of the many reasons I often recommend cognitive-behavioral therapy, since alexithymia may also complicate the psychological processes seen in Somatoneural Dysfunction.

Table 23: DSM-IV Criteria for Posttraumatic Stress Disorder

A. The traumatic event is reexperienced though any of the following:
- Intrusive thought
- Recurrent distressing dreams
- Reliving the event (flashbacks)
- Intense psychological stress or physiological reaction to cues that symbolize the traumatic event

B. Persistent avoidance of stimuli associated with the trauma and numbing of general responsiveness by in three or more of the following ways
- Effort to avoid thoughts or feelings associated with the trauma
- Effort to avoid people or places associated with the trauma
- Inability to recall important aspects of the traums
- Diminished interest in recreational activities
- Feeling of detachment from others
- Restricted range of affect
- Sense of shortened future

C. Persistent symptoms of increased arousal (two or more of the following)
   - Difficulty falling asleep or staying asleep
   - Irritability or outbursts of anger
   - Difficulty concentrating
   - Hypervigilance
   - Exaggerated startle response
D. Duration of symptoms last longer than one month
E. Disturbance causes significant distress or impairment of functioning

In this definition, the traumatic event must involve a threat of serious harm or death to oneself or others nearby and the person's response must Thus it appears that PTSD is not only another subtype of Somatoneural Dysfunction, but may serve as a model to better understand how stress can worsen or even incite the symptoms of SND.

Classically, an event that triggered PTSD was thought to consist of intense fear, helplessness, or horror. It is quite possible, however, that repeated exposure to stressful events of lesser degrees of severity could "add up" to result in a similar complex of symptoms. This may relate back to the "kindling" phenomenon we talked about in regards to multiple chemical sensitivity a few pages back. The duration of symptoms must officially last longer than one month and result in significant impairment of functioning.

Another factor described in PTSD that may apply to Somatoneural Dysfunction in general is that of behavioral conditioning. This theory states that the traumatic event or events become linked with psychological reminders of the trauma. This leads to heightened arousal designed to help avoid re-experiencing the trauma again. A similar conditioned cycle may occur subconsciously with the pain of fibromyalgia, the fatigue of chronic fatigue syndrome, or the perceived "toxic exposures" of multiple chemical sensitivity.

The time course of PTSD can be quite variable. Symptoms may occur as soon as a few days after the inciting event or may not occur until decades later. Symptoms typically wax and wane, often becoming more intense during periods of stress. About 30% of patients recover completely in time, while another 40% show significant improvement in their symptoms (Kaplan and Sadock, 1996).

Successful treatment of PTSD depends on the same methods used to treat other forms of serotonin-deficiency (depression, anxiety, etc). Antidepressants, particularly imipramine and amitriptyline, are the mainstays of medication therapy, while psychotherapy (especially cognitive-behavioral therapy) and other methods of relaxation and stress reduction may be similarly beneficial.

Sleep Disturbances

A close relationship between sleep disturbance and Somatoneural Dysfunction is evident in clinical observation and investigational trials, but is by no means absolute. For a while, researchers thought that some types of SND were primary sleep disorders, with sleep abnormalities as the central inciting event. It hasn't proved that simple, but nonetheless sleep problems play an important role in the development and course of SND in a majority of patients.

Estimates of sleep disruption in fibromyalgia and chronic fatigue syndrome have ranged as high as 95%. Many of these patients have simple insomnia, others have more complex sleep disorders such as narcolepsy or sleep apnea. Non-restorative sleep is virtually universal in SND, but seems to be related to a number of different pathological processes.

Experimental studies done a few decades ago (when regulation of research on human subjects was a bit more lax that it is today) looked at the effects of sleep deprivation both for total sleep time and REM sleep.

Both types of sleep deprivation led to symptoms of fatigue, lack of concentration, lowered pain threshold, headaches, and a host of other complaints that appeared suspiciously like those found in Somatoneural Dysfunction. Military studies were done to study the effects of sleep deprivation on prisoners of war and came up with similar findings.

Alpha-Wave Intrusion

One of the earliest and most striking abnormalities of sleep was discovered in fibromyalgia patients by Moldofsky (1975). These patients had a disruption of stage 4 delta sleep by alpha waves, an EEG pattern resembling that of the waking state. This intrusion was sometimes accompanied by "microarousals" where the patient seemed to be physiologically awake, but had no recollection of the arousal.

Furthermore, artificial disruption of stage 4 sleep by inducing the alpha-wave anomaly with noise leads to development of nonrefreshing sleep and diffuse fatigue and myalgias (Moldofsky, 1976). Once again, the medical profession thought it had stumbled onto the key to Somatoneural Dysfunction, but the rates of this particular sleep anomaly have been highly variable. It may be seen in 50-60% of those with fibromyalgia, 20-30% in chronic fatigue syndrome, 10% in depression, and 5% of normal people.

This was another indication of common disease pathways that led to difficulty in performing studies, mainly because the researchers were all studying different population. What they missed was the fact that this anomaly is seen in a variety of different subtypes of patients all with similar symptoms of fatigue and myalgias. I believe that the vast majority of those "normal" or "depressed" patients had undiagnosed SND due to the mildness of their symptom complex. It also appears that alpha wave intrusion (and to a certain extent, several other types of sleep disorders) may predispose to future development of Somatoneural Dysfunction.

The neurotransmitter serotonin appears to be highest during stage 4 sleep and may be the most important biological factor in sleep regulation. Serotonin plays an important role in the induction of sleep and in maintaining control of its stages. When serotonin levels in the brain rise, sleep is induced. During the rest of the night, serotonin levels fall and rise with the different stages of sleep, being at their highest during the deepest stages of sleep (stages 3 and 4 slow-wave sleep) and at their lowest during REM and alpha activity (Ang, 1999).

It is clear that serotonin also plays a central role in the pathogenesis of Somatoneural Dysfunction due to several observations mentioned previously. It is not certain whether low levels of serotonin lead to decreased slow-wave sleep, or if slow-wave sleep deprivation leads to depressed serotonin activity, however. The most logical possibility is that there is a defect both in the product-ion of serotinin and a decrease in the efficiency of the way the serotonin system works in SND patients.

Table 24: Actions of Serotonin
Sleep Regulation
Mood Elevation
Pain Sensation
Temperature Regulation
Inflammatory Processes
Hormone Regulation
Blood Pressure and Flow

Serotonin also is extremely important in mood. Decreased levels of serotonin are observed in depression, serving as the basis for the treatment of depression with drugs that increase brain levels of serotonin, such as Paxil™.

Serotonin is also essential in setting the sensory pain threshold in the thalamus (Mikkelsson, 1992). Lowered levels contribute to a decreased pain threshold and amplification and processing of normal sensory stimuli as painful or uncomfortable. This can lead to the perception of muscles and joints as swollen or inflamed, as well as an actual neuropathic syndrome of nerve pain and paresthesias.

Blood pressure and flow are also modulated by serotonin release in the blood vessels of the skin and muscles. Temperature control is affected by serotonin levels in the hypothalamus, as well as by its participation in the regulation of blood flow to the body's surface. Lastly, serotonin is an important mediator in the inflammatory and immune cascades.

Patients with Somatoneural Dysfunction have several observable abnormalities from this disturbance in sleep. They awake feeling unrefreshed, often more tired than before they went to sleep. This can be due to overall lack of sleep or lack specifically of enough slow-wave sleep or REM sleep. They commonly have prolonged sleep latency; it takes them longer to fall asleep than normal. They may also wake up several times a night and typically have trouble falling back asleep when they do awaken.

Loss of NREM sleep can result in further serotonin deficiency as well as dysregulation of some of the body's important homeostatic mechanisms. Regulation of adrenal hormone release and immune system control may be altered. The control of the sympathetic nervous system in relation to the fight-or-flight response may be disrupted, leading to increased susceptibility to panic attacks and abnormalities in blood pressure adjustment. The chance of becoming clinically depressed appears to be increased with decreased NREM sleep, and depression in turn, may further worsens other sleep problems itself. Generally, a pervasive feeling of sleepiness and fatigue predominates during the day when duration and quality of sleep declines.

Studies by Moldofsky, mainly in fibromyalgia and chronic fatigue syndrome patients, were able to link sleep disturbance to the symptoms of memory loss and difficulty concentrating. Subjects had impaired performance in mathematical skills, grammar, reasoning, and simple motor tasks. Interestingly, most of the decreased ability was in speed in comp-letion of these tasks, but accuracy was only minimally affected. Patients' own assessments of their performances, however, were sharply reduced (Cote, 1997).

This observation corresponds with a common theme of Somatoneural Dysfunction. Much in the same way that pain is misperceived and amplified and fatigue is focused on by SND patients, there may be a marked amplification of the way they perceive their cognitive function. I have had some patients come to see me because they have had episodes where they forgot where they put their keys or where they parked their cars in a crowded mall. These events, of course, are normal in the range of human cognition and may simply reflect that other thoughts are occupying our minds. A concern of impending Alzheimer's Disease or other neurologic abnormality may occur as well, further contributing to anxiety and depressive symptoms. Increase in pain and fatigue with sleep disturbance seems to be due to a combination of decreased serotonin levels and impaired perception.

Left unchecked, acute sleep deprivation eventually leads to impaired judgment, decreased ability to effectively communicate, neglect of self-care, and impaired performance on tasks requiring motor skills and concentration. Incentive and ability to work declines and periods of "microsleep" or nodding off become more intrusive, resulting in increased tendency for errors and accidents. The same may be true of chronic sleep deprivation.

The effect of REM sleep deprivation is less well understood. Suppression of REM sleep in experimental studies can lead to hyperactivity and impulsivity, symptoms that are uncommon in Somatoneural Dysfunction. Emotional lability (rapid changes in mood), however, may be a symptom of SND that is related to REM sleep deprivation. Chronic REM sleep deprivation has not been adequately studied, but it is likely that this contributes to a decreased ability of the subconscious to interact appropriately to the conscious mind. One theory holds that this may be the root of the dysregulation in control of the immune system, stress, pain, and fatigue symptoms of SND. More research into the function of REM sleep and REM sleep deprivation needs to be done, nonetheless, before any firm conclusions can be made.

Other Sleep Disturbances

Restless leg syndrome or periodic leg movements of sleep (PLMS) is a common problem that may frequently accompany Somatoneural

Dysfunction. Patients may complain of unpleasant aching and drawing sensations in the leg muscles, often associated with a creeping or crawling feeling. These sensations are typically relieved by moving the legs (Krueger, 1990). This syndrome is made worse by fatigue and may produce microarousals that cause overall sleep quality to deteriorate. Sometimes, the patient is even unaware of the symptoms.

Interestingly, these sensations are always classified as painless by medical experts, but PMLS in fibromyalgia patients may be exquisitely painful. Even though some of these "experts" classify this as being related to "hysterical origin", I believe this is simply another instance of pain hypersensitivity in Somatoneural Dysfunction.

Sleep-phase syndrome abnormalities may also occur. The delayed type presents as an inability to fall asleep until 3 to 6 am, with normal awakening occurring at 11 am to 2 pm. An advanced type, with early-evening sleep onset and early-morning awakening also occurs. These syndromes are worsened by shift work, which in my observations almost always serves to worsen SND symptoms.

This may be due, at least in part, to an abnormality in melatonin secretion. Melatonin is a hormone secreted by the pineal gland and is a product of serotonin metabolism. It seems to be important in the regulation of the normal sleep-wake cycle, and indirectly plays a role in the adrenal and gonadal systems. Its main role is in adjusting day-night rhythms and may become disordered by jet lag or with a change in shift work schedule. Patients with Somatoneural Dysfunction appear to be more susceptible to melatonin dysregulation.

Narcolepsy has been given a distasteful connotation in the media. For some reason it was thought comical for a person to be affected with an overwhelming desire to sleep, and narcoleptics were thus portrayed as buffoons or mental patients. Classically speaking, narcolepsy is a disabling disorder of sleep attacks and muscle paralysis (cataplexy). Fortunately, this severe form of narcolepsy is actually quite rare.

Much more common is "independent narcolepsy" or essential hypersomnolence, which is characterized by a distressing pattern of daytime sleepiness that interferes with school, work, or social situations. The cause of both types of narcolepsy is related to REM onset. In true narcoleptics, REM sleep seems to intrude upon normal wakefulness, and is accompanied by greatly reduced sleep latency. In essential hypersomnolence, a deficiency in nighttime REM sleep leads to REM rebound during the day and difficulty in staying awake. Patients with Somatoneural Dysfunction and its associated REM sleep disturbance are prone to this hypersomnolence.

Sleep-disordered breathing, or sleep apnea, may also play a role in Somatoneural Dysfunction. Sleep apnea syndrome results when a decreased level of oxygen in the brain leads to microarousals that interfere with sleep. This also leads to poor concentration, memory disturbances, daytime sleepiness, fatigue, and aches and pains that are worse in the morning and with inactivity.

Sleep apnea in association with SND is partially central and partially obstructive. Central sleep apnea generally occurs as a result of injury to the areas of the brain that control the process of respiration. The brain controls respiration via outflow from the autonomic nervous system. It is this part of the process that may be altered in SND. Dysregulation of the autonomic nervous system leads to decrease in the ventilatory drive during sleep and is accompanied by retained carbon dioxide and lower levels of oxygen in the bloodstream.

Obstructive sleep apnea is most often related to excess tissue in the back of the throat. This tissue may fall back and obstruct the airway, causing snoring and decreased oxygenation. In SND, sleep apnea may also be related to deconditioned respiratory musculature or defects in the neurologic control of breathing during certain stages of sleep, particularly REM and slow-wave sleep. The sleep disruption in patients with Somatoneural Dysfunction may thus be related to a combination of factors. Primary sleep disturbances should always be sought and treated if present.

Chapter 6:
Diet

Recommendations for a healthy diet low in saturated fat and cholesterol and maintenance near ideal body weight and lean body mass are generalities that hold true for all patients. This, unfortunately, is much easier said than done. A diet consisting of 18% protein, 52% fat, and 30% carbohydrates has been shown to be healthy, promote weight loss, and help to control symptoms of chronic fatigue. In this section I will describe this dietary approach, as well as pointing out some factors that may be a part of Somatoneural Dysfunction and necessitate special dietary techniques. These factors include irritable bowel syndrome, gastroesophageal reflux disease, and reactive hypoglycemia.

There are a ton (pardon the pun) of diets out there, in addition to barrels of dietary substitutes and supplements purported to promote weight loss. Most of them are safe and some are even effective. Any reasonable diet may be effective in SND, but should probably be monitored by a registered dietician at the initiation. This will prevent trying "fad" diets with possible adverse health effects. And remember, any diet pill that says "take this "Super Fat Away Plus" diet pill with a big glass of water and watch the fat roll away", will not help you lose weight. The big glass of water, however, may fill you up and help you lose a few pounds in that manner. Also, read the fine print on those things. Most require a low-calorie diet and rigorous exercise program in addition to Super Fat Away Plus. Save your money. Buy more copies of this book instead!

One of the most popular diets, called the "Zone Diet", has been adopted by many patients with fibromyalgia and chronic fatigue without any real evidence that it works. This diet, proposed by Sears and Lawren (Sears, 1995) claims that the ideal dietary ratio of fat to protein to carbo-hydrate is 30:30:40. By doing this, you would optimize insulin to glucagon balance and thus eicosanoid production. Eicosanoids are, according to Dr. Sears, the root of all disease, and control of their produc-tion to allow "good eicosanoids" to outweigh "bad eicosanoids" will allow you to improve your immune function, increase your energy level, enhance mental clarity, and facilitate peak athletic performance. I think the good eicosanoids will also paint your house with tiny little paint-brushes if you ask them nicely.

Amazingly, this diet has come to such widespread use without a shred of evidence to support its use. Many of the theories proposed in the Zone Diet have been proven wrong. Sears claims that insulin is the culprit for producing "bad eicosanoids", and by reducing insulin production with a low carbohydrate diet, "bad eicosanoids" can be minimized. If that were so simple and true, juvenile-onset diabetics (who have little or no insulin) should be the healthiest people around. With low levels of insulin, one would have high levels of glucose, which is bad (unless one considers accelerated atherosclerosis, heart attacks, blindness, neuropathy, and kid-ney failure good).

What is important in this theory is not so much eicosanoids (which are really metabolites of essential fatty acids), but the essential fatty acids themselves, which we can only get from the foods we eat, and can be manipulated in our diet.

Another point of the Zone Diet is growth hormone production enhancement, which is thought to be beneficial in maintaining health.

Unfortunately, no evidence has been found to suggest that the diet does anything to affect growth hormone production. Dr. Sears bases his findings on studies involving the injection of subjects with human growth hormone! Excess growth hormone causes a condition called acromegaly, or gigantism, which, in addition to making you look odd, can lead to liver and kidney failure.

A recent article published in <u>Sports Medicine</u> debunks the zone myth of the diet leading to enhanced exercise performance by allowing increased blood flow to the muscles by producing a certain eicosanoid. Actually, the particular eicosanoid Sears speaks of is not even found in skeletal muscle, and no evidence in human trials has found significant increases of blood flow at biologic doses (Cheuvront, 1997). Interestingly, the diet also claims to enhance athletic performance without benefit of exercise, a ridiculous notion.

In addition, the Zone Diet recommends a much higher concentration of fat and protein than any national organization, which base their findings on scientific study, not anecdotes and outdated theories. It also eliminates bread, cereals, and grains, which have been shown to be beneficial in reducing some types of cancers and in supplying important nutrients, vitamins, and minerals. The diet is, however, calorie deficient. You will lose weight on the Zone Diet, which may be why some patients report feeling better. I believe there are easier, safer, and more effective ways to do it, however, and that the Zone Diet offers no special advantages over other calorie-deficient diets.

Another problem I have with the Zone Diet is the restrictions, and this illustrates a point I like to make about diets. The only snacks allowed in the zone are fruit, cottage cheese, low fat yogurt, and low fat milk. That's it. Ever. This ignores the important concept that eating is enjoyable and partly dependant on variety. Personally, I would rather have all my fingernails pulled out than eat yogurt and cottage cheese for the rest of my life.

The popularity of the Zone Diet illustrates how things make their way from the medical field to general use. Some physician or researcher develops a theory that may or may not make any sense. It generally takes about 3-4 years to get the theory out to the public. During that time, other researchers disprove the original theory. There is then a 3-4 year window that occurs between those two occurrences and the general populace believes that the four-year old theory is true, when in fact it has already been disproven. The marketers spend a lot of money on advertisements, some well-known Hollywood people use the diet, and you have an instant fad.

In Somatoneural Dysfunction, however, such a diet may result in nutritional deficiencies that actually worsen pain, fatigue, and exercise tolerance in the long run, once the euphoria of weight loss resolves. Besides, certainly not all SND patients are overweight and would not benefit from such caloric restriction.

As an alternative, I recommend a diet similar to the DASH diet. DASH stands for "Dietary Approaches to Stop Hypertension" and consists of whole grains, poultry, fish, and nuts with emphasis on fruits, vegetables and low-fat dairy products. Fats, red meats, sweets, and sugar-containing beverages are reduced. The combination was approximately 55% carbohydrates, 27% fats, and 18% protein. Fats were further divided into saturated (6%), monounsaturated (13%), and polyunsaturated (8%).

Target levels for other nutrients differ only slightly in the SND Diet. This comes out to approximately no more than 2 servings of fish, meat, or poultry, 7 to 8 servings of grains, 4 to 5 servings of fruit, 2 to 3servings of low-fat dairy products, 4 to 5 vegetable servings per day and 4 to 5 servings of nuts or legumes per week. The DASH diet not only significantly lowered blood pressure in hypertensive patients, but resulted in a 50% improvement in patient reported quality of life when compared to the control diet (Plaisted, 1999).

Table 25: Nutrient Targets

Nutrient	Target	DASH
Cholesterol	150	150
Potassium	4566	4566
Magnesium	600	484
Calcium	1500	1200
Sodium	3000	3000

The carbohydrate/protein/fat ratio used in the DASH diet appears to have a beneficial effect on mood and performance, even in an "at-risk" population such as night-shift workers (Paz, 1997), but does seem to have several drawbacks. Higher amounts of carbohydrates and fats are needed for peak exercise performance and mood, respectively (Maughan, 1997, Wells, 1998). Therefore, I suggest that meal composition be altered throughout the day and throughout the workweek to align more closely with the body's natural circadian rhythms and take into account the burdens of modern life.

Breakfast recommendations are higher in carbohydrate content to allow for more energy to start the day. Lunches are higher in fat to keep mood elevated. This is particularly important on-the-job, where stress can decrease mood and concentration. Dinner would be higher in carbohydrates again, as well as slightly higher in protein to allow for exercise and subsequent relaxation. The beginning of the week should allow for more liberal caloric intake, increasing through the middle of the week, and declining as weekend approaches.

Total caloric intake should be dependant on the lean body mass to allow for weight loss or weight maintenance as needed. The guidelines and recommendations at the end of this chapter are meant to give approximation of the program. Specific meal plans and dietary implementation should take place under the guidance of a registered dietician. There are lots of them around and they're generally a great resource that is usually a fully covered benefit with most health insurance plans. More specific information on the DASH diet can also be found at http://www.nhlbi.nih.gov/health/public/heart/hbp/dash/. Free copies can be requested at this site.

Other healthy diets include the Mediterranean diet, the AHA/NCEP diet (American Heart Association/National Cholesterol Education Program), and the Dean Ornish healthy heart diet. The Mediterranean diet recommends spare use of red meat and dairy products, and small portions of fish, eggs, and poultry are eaten several times each week. Olive oil or canola oil is the primary sources of fats, while grains, fresh fruits, and vegetable account for the majority of calories. The AHA/NCEP diet is similar to the DASH diet, but has slightly lower protein and higher fat contents. The Ornish diet is a vegetarian program that limits fat intake to less than 10%. Each of these approaches has some data to suggest beneficial effects on reducing the risk of such illness as cancer and cardiovascular disease (Pinkowish, 1999). The diet that follows takes the best recommendations for general health from each of these approaches.

Two additional general dietary strategies that have been found useful in health maintenance and in chronic fatigue have been supplementation with ω-3 fatty acids, and reduction of polyunsaturated fat to saturated fat ratio to less than 2 to 1. The ω-3 fatty acids are generally found in fish and fish oils and have been long suspected to promote good health and longevity.

Special Diet Circumstances

Bowel dysfunction is an all-too-common part of Somatoneural Dysfunction and sometimes necessitates a slightly different approach to dietary management. These abnormalities fall into several symptom complexes: irritable bowel, hypoglycemia, reactive hypoglycemia, or gastroesophageal reflux disease.

Hypoglycemia

Hypoglycemic patients typically get lightheaded or dizzy after not eating for several hours. The reason why this appears to be such a mysterious ailment both among patients and doctors eludes me. In my practice, if a patient feels they are getting some unusual symptoms when they are fasting I ask them to spend a day with me to figure it out. I ask them not to eat anything after midnight and come to my office at 8 am. They are then free to peruse my extensive collection of Sports Illustrated™ or Redbook™

until they begin to feel their usual symptoms. I then measure their blood sugars. Below 70 indicates that they are getting hypoglycemic symptoms, it's that simple.

The body is designed to maintain blood glucose at most any cost and will release glucagon (kind of the opposite to insulin in the hormone world) in order to kickstart the glucose-making process in the liver and release some of the stored glucose in the body. Usually, in hypoglycemic patients, this system doesn't work right. Occasionally, excess insulin is to blame, so insulin levels should be measured in all cases of documented hypoglycemia.

If the patient's glucose is normal, I have them wait another hour and draw another sample. If it is still normal, I have them eat and look for other causes of their symptoms. If nothing else is found, I look for other signs and symptoms of SND as the symptoms can be another manifestation of this syndrome. Everyone gets neuropsychiatric symptoms at a certain time of fasting, from lightheadedness and giddiness all the way to hallucinations and fainting. For most this takes days, or even weeks given the strength of an individual's compensatory mechanisms. In SND, this system is defective and unable to hold off symptoms for as little as a few hours during the day.

Typical dietary management of hypoglycemia of this type is merely eating smaller, more frequent meals. Snacks should consist of a combination of sweet foods with rapidly absorbed glucose (grapes, strawberries, raisins) and high protein/carbohydrate items (granola bars, yogurt). Vegetables such as carrots and celery are essentially "free" and should be used even between snacks if symptoms are present. An increase in the carbohydrate to protein ratio of the DASH diet can also reduce hypoglycemic symptoms, but will often result in unacceptable weight gain.

In patients with reactive hypoglycemia, symptoms typically occur one to two hours after meals. This results from a hypersensitivity to insulin release that occurs after meals, and leads to abnormally low glucose levels. There may also be an abnormality in the usual balance between glucagon and insulin that is responsible for regulating blood glucose levels. This type of hypoglycemia is detected with a Oral Glucose Tolerance Test (OGTT), which has the patient drink a carbohydrate solution and then measures blood glucose levels at one, two, and three hours afterwards. Patients with reactive hypoglycemia will show a characteristic drop in glucose level instead of the usual peak and gradual decline.

Treatment for hypoglycemia consists of eating higher carbohydrate meals or adding snacks two hours after each meal. Weight gain is an obvious problem for these patients, but a good nutritionist can outline a high carbohydrate meal plan that is relatively low in calories. Occasionally, medications are required to blunt the abnormal sensitivity to insulin and rebalance the insulin/glucagon ratio.

Irritable Bowel Syndrome

Simply stated, patients with IBS should avoid foods that make their symptoms worse. Yes, for this I spent nearly a decade in medical training! Actually, this approach can be harder than in sounds and often takes a meticulously kept food diary to sort out what foods worsen the disorder. In general, three groups of foods are the most common culprits in exacerbating IBS: dairy products, sweeteners, or legumes.

Lactose intolerance is present in a great deal of IBS patients and there is significant overlap between the two syndromes in symptomatology, therapy, and course. Lactose is a type of carbohydrate found in dairy products that is similar to glucose, but requires an enzyme called lactase to digest and utilize. I suggest a trial of a lactose-free diet (where again, the help of a registered dietician can be very helpful) for all patients with significant IBS symptoms.

Sorbitol and fructose are similar sugars that may also produce symptoms if a patient lacks the required enzyme. These are most commonly found as artificial sweeteners and should be avoided whenever possible. Interestingly, all of these enzyme deficiencies may develop in childhood or much later in life depending on whether the deficiency is inherited or acquired. Nuts and seeds are to be avoided in IBS and other gastrointestinal ailments such as diverticulosis.

Gastroesophageal Reflux Disease (GERD)

Weakness in the lower esophageal sphincter (LES) may allow acid from the stomach to reflux back up into the esophagus. When this becomes symptomatic, the syndrome of GERD develops. Acid belongs in the stomach, as it has a protective lining and prostaglandin coating. It does not, of course, belong in the esophagus.

Acid in the esophagus may result in a spectrum of symptoms attributable to the direct irritation of the upper gastrointestinal and respiratory tract or from the body's attempt at ridding itself of the offending acid. The typical sensation of heartburn is usually, but not always present and occurs when inflammation of the lining of the esophagus occurs. Regurgitation of stomach contents (yum!) is sometimes present if the weakness of the LES is particularly severe.

Acid is also irritating to the larynx and vocal cords. Inflammation in these places may result in chronic dry cough, hoarseness, or the sensation of something stuck in the throat. This symptom used to be called "globus hystericus" because doctors would look down into their patient's throats and see nothing to cause difficulty swallowing. They then suspected the patients were crazy. At some point some smart throat doctors discovered what was really going on and allowed for treatment of this annoying condition.

Another entity that can cause symptoms ranging from annoying to severe is esophageal spasm. When acid refluxes back into the esophagus and causes irritation, the esophagus fights back. Unfortunately, the only method of defense the poor esophagus has is spasm. This is actually the main line of defense for most organs in the body when something is irritating or gets stuck (like kidney stones or gallstones). The esophagus essentially tries to squeeze the acid back down into the stomach where it belongs. Regrettably, this squeezing process is painful and has sent many a patient rushing to the local emergency room thinking they were having a heart attack.

For patients with symptoms of heartburn or GERD, some additional dietary guidelines should be followed. Most importantly, elimination of alcohol, caffeine, and chocolate should commence, since these items reduce LES pressure. No eating should be done within an hour of bedtime and care should be taken to avoid overeating. Smoking also lowers the LES pressure and is another reason to quit. In case you didn't realize it, I'll let you in on a little secret: smoking is bad for you!

The Somatoneural Dysfunction Diet

Poultry, fish, and vegetables are the mainstay of the SND diet and account for six servings per day. Serving size varies, but approximates 3 ounces of cooked fish or poultry, a half cup cooked vegetables, or a cup of raw vegetables. Remember to use primarily ocean fish. Fish like catfish, trout, and salmon are usually raised on "fish farms" and are essentially big fat fish. We want to eat lean, mean, fighting fish. Poultry generally means chicken or turkey, but Cornish game hen, duck, or game birds can be substituted as long as they are trimmed of fat and skinned. Vegetables, particularly green, leafy ones, are rich in magnesium and B vitamins. Red meat is discouraged, but can be substituted 2-3 times a week if desired, as long as portion size is kept to 3 ounces and trimmed of all fat.

Grains are the usual sources of fiber and carbohydrates. They are used liberally in both the DASH and Mediterranean diets, but I recommend only four servings per day in order to help maintain ideal body weight or promote weight loss. Grain snacks (such as popcorn, wheat crackers, or unsalted pretzels), however, may be spread liberally throughout the day in 3-4 servings.

I recommend limiting or eliminating nuts and seeds entirely due to detrimental effect on GI function. Instead, one serving of beans per day (or 3-4 times a week) can be substituted. Beans are an underutilized source of fiber, magnesium, potassium, and energy and can be used as a side dish or part of a main meal.

Increasing fruit in the diet is often a difficult chore for Americans for some reason. One serving of fruit (one medium fresh fruit, half cup of fruit juice, or a half cup of canned fruit) should accompany each meal, while two additional servings are allowed as snacks through the day. Almost any fruit will do and will vary according to each person's preferences, but bulkier items like apples, bananas, oranges, or peaches tend to be more filling with meals than raisins, grapes, dates, or prunes. The latter should be reserved for snacking. Remember to limit serving sizes to a half-cup in any event. My mother once went on a "Watermelon Diet" that said you could eat as much watermelon as you wanted. She proceeded to eat a whole watermelon every day and needless to say, did not lose any weight. She actually began to look like a watermelon, but that's another story.

Dairy products are high in calcium and protein, but also tend to be high in fat. Three servings a day are recommended, but extra care must be taken to choose only very low fat or fat free items. Even "fat free" frozen yogurt can have a lot of calories, so should be further limited. Eight ounces of milk, a cup of yogurt, or one ounce of cheese make up a serving.

Fats and oils are generally used in cooking or as condiments and can be a hidden source of calories. One serving is all that is allowed with each meal and includes one teaspoon of vegetable oil (olive oil is recommended), two tablespoons of lowfat salad dressing, or one teaspoon of butter or margarine.

The DASH diet recommends sweets as snacks, but I am both more liberal and more strict in my guidelines. Sweets like gelatin, hard candies, maple syrup, and jelly beans are allowed by DASH, but add little nutritionally to the diet and should be avoided. I sacrifice calories to allow the addition of "pleasure foods". One serving of cookies, cake, pie, whatever, is allowed per day, as long as three hundred calories are not exceeded.

Table 26: Diet Overview			
Food Group	Examples	Serving Size	Daily Servings
1) Fish/Poultry	chicken, turkey, tuna	3 oz.	0-6
2) Vegetables	potatoes, carrots, peas	½-1 cup	0-6
3) Grains	bread, cereal, rice	1 slice-1/2 cup	4
4) Fruits	apples, bananas, pears	½ cup-1 fruit	5
5) Dairy (low fat)	milk, cheese, yogurt	½ cup	3
6) Fats/oils	butter, oil, salad dressing	1 tsp-1 tbsp	3
7) Snacks	cookies, cake, chocolate	less than 300 cal.	1

Tricks and Hints

1) Some food categories don't fit in with the ones above. Eggs or pasta could be substituted for fish/poultry or vegetable, but should be limited to three times a week each. One egg or one cup of pasta equals one serving.

2) Portion control is essential to any diet. If you are a big eater, 3 ounces of chicken can go down in one bite. The key is to use meat/fish/poultry as part of the entrée and not as the whole meal. Soups and stews are an excellent way to make a few ounces of meat go a long way. Crockpot cooking has become my own personal way to enjoy tasty, easy-to-prepare foods that are healthy and low in calories.

3) If you have trouble sticking to the diet, ease into it gradually. Adjust portion size and number of servings by a little each week.

4) Remember that the type of food is more important than the calo-
    ries. If you are maintaining a healthy weight, you can be as liberal
    as you want with the portion size and number of servings. A
    healthy, six-foot five-inch guy may weight two-hundred and forty
    pounds and will require a good deal more than the two thousand
    or so calories this diet suggests.

5) Space the snacks throughout the day and make sure that you meas-
    ure them out beforehand. Don't sit down with a bag of potato
    chips and think that you're only going to eat 5 chips. Substitute
    things like pickles or rice cakes, which are very low in calories and
    very healthy.

6) Keep track of what you eat. A food diary is one of the most helpful
    things you can do.

7) If you slip, get right back on track when you can. Everyone slips
    and food is a pleasurable part of life. You should not feel guilty
    about the occasional chicken wing outburst or hot fudge fiasco on
    occasion. Try and minimize these episodes and they won't have as
    much of an impact on your overall diet.

Several cookbooks are excellent resources for making tasty dishes that
fit in nicely with this program and include:
1) The Mediterranean Diet Cookbook: A Delicious Alternative
    for Lifelong Health. Nancy Harmon Jenkins and Antonia
    Trichopoulou. Bantam Books. 1994
2) The Mediterranean Herb Cookbook: Fresh and Savory
    Recipes from the Mediterranean Garden. Georgeann
    Brennan. Chronicle. 2000.
3) Everyday Cooking with Dr. Dean Ornish: 150 Easy Low-Fat,
    High Flavor Recipes. Dean Ornish, MD. HarperTrade. 1997.

Chapter 7:
Exercise

Well, now this is certainly a challenge. How can I tell my patients, who don't feel good, who are tired, and who ache all over, to go out and exercise. I do it like this: "Go out and exercise! Now!"

I will be a little more specific in outlining an exercise treatment plan, but that principle remains key. Too many of the populist books ignore the beneficial effects of exercise on their patients simply because it is hard to get patients to do it. People make excuses why they can't exercise and I've listed the top ten and my typical responses below.

Top Five Reasons Why Patients with SND Cannot Exercise

#5: "I don't have the time…"   My program takes four and a half hours a week, 10-20 minutes each night during the week and an hour each night of the weekend. While I realize that people are busy, everyone can spare this much time to improve their health. Turn off the TV and send the kids to grandmas, everyone will understand why you will need this time for yourself. In the long run, staying healthy will give you much more time to enjoy the good things in life, so time to exercise will never be time wasted.

#4: "I don't have the energy…"   Most patients with SND are deconditioned and will have a hard time starting an exercise program. I realize this. This is part of what we're fighting against. This is something that must be overcome. Patients must push themselves to do this and will find that with time and consistency it gets easier and easier.

#3: "I can't, it hurts…"   I realize this also. After a thorough physical and laboratory examination by a physician experienced in exercise programs for SND, we should be relatively sure that such a program will not cause any harm. Abnormalities of bone and disorders of metabolism and muscle will have been ruled out and cardiovascular risk factors will have been assessed. Any patient with more than two cardiac risk factors and a sedentary life style for over six months should have a stress test to assure cardiovascular competence. If all is well, start the program. If you're sore afterwards, use ice or heating pads or other techniques described later to limit the pain and discomfort. If necessary, decrease the time of exercise by a few minutes and gradually work up to the recommended time. Most important is to hang in there and keep trying!

Table 27: Cardiac Risk Factors
• Family history of premature heart disease in close relatives(<55 in females, <45 in males)
• Diabetes
• Hyperlipidemia
• Hypertension
• Smoking
• Male sex or postmenopause in females

#2: "Exercise is boring…"   So is feeling miserable and not being able to do some of the things that make life fun. There are many ways to make exercise less dull, including adding a lot of variation to your routine and engaging in competitive activities to keep things interesting

#1: "I'm not very good at exercising..."   Nobody says you have to be good. This is one case where just doing it is good enough to gain all of the benefits.

The Program

So, now that we have dealt with all the reasons not to exercise, you are ready to go! I divide these approaches into two types: the home exercise program and formal physical therapy. I usually start patients with a home program due to convenience, but progress rapidly to a competent physical therapy program if there is no initial response to the home program or the symptoms appear particularly severe.

Often, patients are told not to exercise by family, friends, or even physicians for fear of worsening symptoms or causing some harm. Some studies have erroneously concluded that exercise programs were not of any benefit, but this is due to high dropout rates of participants. Obviously, it is not easy for people who spend so much time being tired and achy to get up and exercise, but it is crucial in dealing with this disorder. Numerous studies have shown the benefits of exercise in patients with Somatoneural Dysfunction. One trial showed that chronically fatigued patients, even those with

> I tell patients they are like an NFL running back who has suffered a severe knee injury. He can sit back and watch a million dollar career go down the drain, or he can get out there and fight through the pain in order to get back in the starting lineup....

severely debilitating illnesses, could tolerate thirty minutes a day of intermittent light exercise without exacerbating their symptoms (Durstine, 2000). An excellent British study in chronic fatigue syndrome showed a marked improvement in functional work capacity and fatigue in patients given a graded exercise program (Powell, 2001).

In fibromyalgia, short term studies have been done to show the safety and efficacy of exercise (Meiworm, 2000), but longer term follow-up is still lacking. I base my recommendations on a trial done in Canada a few years ago, which utilized a combination of aerobic exercise, flexibility, and strengthening (Martin, 1996). They were able to demonstrate a dramatic reduction in pain from tender points at the end of the program.

Furthermore, the other benefits of exercise are well known: cardiovascular health and enhanced sense of well being are the most important, but there are numerous others so, read on. We are just beginning to realize how regular exercise affects the physiology and pathophysiology of the human body.

Table 28: General Health Benefits of Exercise

Reduction in the risk of heart attack and stroke

Improvement in blood flow

Reduction in total cholesterol and LDL
Blood pressure reduction
Decreased risk of certain cancers (colon, uterus, prostate, breast)
Reduce the risk of diabetes and control elevated glucose levels
Control weight and prevent obesity
Increase bone mass and reduce the risk of osteoporosis
Prevent pain by improving back strength, endurance, and mobility
Reverse age-related decline in aerobic fitness and respiratory function
Promote self-confidence, increased energy, and well being, possibly by
    enhancing release of ß-endorphin and increasing levels of serotonin
    in the brain

My Program

The following is a program I have found useful for a variety of patients from 14-94 years old and in all types of physical condition. Emphasis is on variety to prevent boredom, flexibility to improve muscle and joint dynamics, and strengthening to protect against fatigue. In Somatoneural Dysfunction, the body is not able to effectively deal with stressors such as pain and fatigue, so we strengthen everything else.

Day 1 is on Monday. Most of life's challenges start on Monday. I begin with a 20-minute program designed to enhance energy for the rest of the week's endeavors. Flexibility training is emphasized here using either tai chi or yoga techniques. In one of the few documented studies done on tai chi, in Australia in the late 1980s, researchers demonstrated that tai chi could increase heart rate, alter cortisol secretion, and enhance norepinephrine production in ways similar to a moderate exercise program. Practitioners found that they experienced "less tension, depression, anger, fatigue, confusion and state-anxiety, they felt more vigorous, and in general they had less mood disturbance" than non-practitioners (Jin, 1989).

Yoga has for centuries been used in Eastern medical practices for pain control and treatment of fatigue states. A British trial from 1993 showed that pranayama (yogic breathing and stretch) could produce an increase in perceptions of mental and physical energy, enthusiasm, and alertness (Wood, 1993). Others studies have looked at yoga in control of painful symptoms of problems like carpal tunnel (Garfinkel, 1998) and osteoarthritis of the hands (Garfinkel, 1994). It also enhances flexibility, stamina, and endurance.

These sessions are best taught by an experienced practitioner. I have found that group sessions are most beneficial, both in enhancing outcome and compliance with the regimen. Once a patient is comfortable with the program, they may progress to an individual home-based program if more convenient. Most health maintenance organizations offer Tai Chi and/or yoga classes for their patients, while others may find groups at local health clubs, colleges, or community organizations for reasonable rates.

Flexibility training also reduces the risk of subsequent musculoskeletal injury, even if it only consists of range-of-motion stretches. Therefore, in addition to Monday's routine, range-of-motion stretching of all major muscle and tendon groups should be done prior to each day's exercise. Feldenkreis or Alexander techniques are excellent places to start and can be taught by skilled practitioners. More information on these methods is available under the physical therapy section in volume 2.

Day 2, Tuesday, should allow for a more intensive aerobic workout, but for only a short duration. The type of program is less important than its ability to get your heart rate up and get you sweating for ten minutes. This can be done with swimming, brisk walking, aerobic dance, bicycling, rollerblading, or any similar activity. For patients who are particularly deconditioned or who have other limiting medical problem (emphysema, rheumatoid arthritis, congestive heart failure) a gentle walk may suffice. It may be necessary at first to decrease the time of exercise if ten minutes results in exhaustion or extreme pain. In that case, start at one minute and increase by a minute each week until the goal is met. It is important to set aside the required time for yourself, prepare for the exercise and complete what you set out to do. Recovery from Somatoneural Dysfunction is a marathon, not a sprint.

Aerobic training should be initiated at a target heart rate of 55% of age predicted maximum heart rate (defined as 220 beats per minute minus the person's age). As conditioning increases over time, the target heart rate should also increase, to a maximum of 80% of the age predicted maximum. Exercise should be kept at a moderate intensity level, particularly with sessions longer than ten minutes. Someone engaged in moderate-intensity exercise should be able to carry on a conversation (Trotto, 1999).

Don't forget that stretching exercises should be done in preparation for all activities recommended here. All major muscle groups should be gently stretched prior to exercise, starting from the hands/wrists and feet/ankles through to the back and neck. When finished, the same set of stretches should be done again, after a "cool down" period of leisurely walking.

Wednesday is the third day and should consist of a strengthening program and last an average of twenty minutes. For beginners or elderly patients, this can be as simple as adding one-pound weights to your ankles and wrists and going for a walk. Even that little bit extra can add dramatically to strength and endurance. For more conditioned patients, the strengthening program is probably best served with nautilus equipment at a community center or health club. A nautilus circuit is designed to strengthen each muscle group individually. Start with whatever setting you can do easily for ten repetitions. Each week add two more repetitions until you reach twenty comfortably, then go up one notch in resistance.

For patients who are very deconditioned or in a lot of pain, the exercises done with the nautilus equipment can be simulated without using the equipment. If you are working the bench press machine, simply lie on the bench and pretend you are doing bench presses with weights. This will work very well to begin to retrain the muscles, bones, and joints to prepare them for strengthening and conditioning.

For those without access to such equipment, I typically refer to a physical therapy center for a three or four week course. Good programs are able to set up each patient with home programs for strengthening at the end of this time period without the need for buying expensive equipment.

Such resistance training has favorable effects on blood pressure, lipid levels, glucose tolerance, cardiovascular function, and bone mineral density (Pollock, 1996). Even in frail elderly patients between the ages of 80 and 90, remarkable gains can be seen. Increases of over 100% in muscle strength have been noted over as little as 10 weeks, in addition to dramatic improvements in balance and decrease in falls (Fiatarone, 1994).

Thursday is a day for a light competitive workout. Competition adds some excitement and interest to the program and makes things fun. Generally, this necessitates finding a partner to compete against. In my practice, I pair up patients with Somatoneural Dysfunction for this activity, which seems to enhance the overall success of the experience. Sports are usually the activities for Thursday and can range from more intense activities such as racquetball or basketball, to moderate activities like tennis, to light sports like badminton, table tennis, or even darts. Leisure sports such as golf and bowling can be substituted, but obviously take a good deal longer. The important part of Thursday activity is to engage in constructive competition, which enhances a sense of well-being and provides mental as well as physical challenge to everyone involved. Anything where you actually move a little bit and keep the mind involved is worthwhile to start. I have one patient who is 92 and limited in her daily activities by emphysema. I have her play checkers or canasta, and keep telling her the important thing is to keep playing. She still beats me at checkers, by the way.

Table 29: Sample Week of Exercises	
Monday	Flexibility Training (yoga, stretching, tai chi)
	• 20 minutes
Tuesday	Aerobic Exercise (aerobics, bicycling, running/walking)
	• 10 minutes
Wednesday	Strength Training (Nautilus™, free weights, isometrics)
	• 20 minutes
Thursday	Light Competitive
	• 10 minutes or more
Friday	Endurance Training (any of the four types of exercise)
	• 60 minutes
Saturday	Heavy Competitive
	• 60 minutes
Sunday	REST

Fridays and Saturdays are the days I recommend the most intensive periods of exercise. They are generally times when you don't have to work the next day, which allows added "recovery time". If you work on weekends, adjust this schedule so that the longest exercise days fall before a day off. The first long day should be used for aerobic exercise, while the second should consist of a more competitive workout. Sunday is, of course, a day of rest. Some examples of each type of workout were alluded to earlier in this section and can be found in the following tables, along with a summary of a typical week in the program.

The following activities are listed in order of exercise capacity needed to complete, i.e. most strenuous first, down to the least strenuous. Pick one that you enjoy and that you can accomplish without overstraining. Some require specialized equipment or facilities, while others can be done at home. Many may require partners as well. Consideration should also be given to expense while selecting activities. I have given several options that should be free or of minimal expense, but encourage my patients to keep in mind that $40-50 for membership in a health club or gym is a relatively modest sum to pay when compared to the overall cost of health care. If we can prevent one day in the hospital or one emergency room visit, the cost of a year's membership is covered. Also, patients should read some of the fine print on their managed care contracts as most organizations offer discounts at many local clubs and events. Or, if you happen to be fabulously wealthy, a personal trainer can be extremely helpful in all types of activities. And remember to buy several more copies of this book as well...

The times listed are for frame of reference only and constitute the "goal" regimen. Obviously, most patients will not be able to do sixty-minute workouts at first. Each patient should participate in a given activity for as long as they feel comfortably when first beginning. If they have to, I tell patients to start at one minute and increase by a minute every few days. However, that doesn't mean you should spend one minute on a treadmill and then go sit on your couch and eat bonbons all night. Stay in the gym, watch others exercise, visualize yourself exercising. This will condition your mind to accept an exercise regimen as part of the necessary road back to health. The mind, remember, needs to be conditioned as much as the body.

Table 30: Types of Activities

Flexibility	Aerobic	Strength	Competitive
Tai-Chi	Running	Free Weights	Skiing
Yoga	Aerobics	Nautilus	Racquetball
Stretching	Swimming	Wrestling	Basketball
Qi-gong	Rollerblading	Boxing	Tennis
Range of Motion	Stair Climbing	Isometrics	Golf
	Rowing		Bowling
	Backpacking		Badminton
	Dancing		Table Tennis
	Frisbee		Croquet
	Fishing		Billiards

Tai chi is a traditional Chinese martial art that uses slow and graceful movements to relax body and mind. Practitioners believe it to promote blood circulation, loosen tight joints, tone the muscles, decreases nervous system irritability, and promote cardiovascular health. It also benefits concentration, coordination, and balance. These potential benefits make it the ideal flexibility program for patients with Somatoneural Dysfunction, particularly those who are quite deconditioned or elderly.

Yoga, Qui-gong, and stretching are variations on a similar theme, utilizing mechanical stretching, breathing, and meditation to provide both physical and mental strengthening. Yoga, as taught over centuries in the practice of Ayurvedic Medicine, involves a series of body positions and movements along with meditation and breathing exercises that relax the mind and body. Qui-gong (of which T'ai chi is one style) involves breathing, meditation, and stationary and moving exercises to focus the body's energy. Range of motion is simply putting each joint and muscle group through its typical full range of motion against the resistance of gravity for the least strenuous workout for flexibility.

Aerobics may be of any type: dance, step, or any of the common variations. Free weights entail use of barbells at a gym or at home, while nautilus utilizes resistance machines that work individual muscle groups in turn. The rest of the activities listed should be self-explanatory.

Isometrics is the practice of engaging one muscle group against another. It thus has a very broad range of energy expenditure because it is directly proportional to the amount exerted. For example, if you place both hands in front of you resting against your chest and press them against each other, you can control the amount of force applied. The amount of energy expended is proportional to the strength of each individual person and thus can be useful even in those who are quite elderly or debilitated as well as weightlifters and bodybuilders.

Summary

There are several important points to remember about exercise programs. First of all, everyone must recognize how important this is. I really cannot expect anyone to get better without putting in the minimal effort required here to strengthen the body. At maximum this takes 3-4 hours per week and there are no excuses

Second, it doesn't really matter the type of activity you engage in. I've given some examples in the previous pages, but the rest is up to you. Stretch, sweat, strengthen, and start slow. Whether it is completing a triathalon or playing tiddlywinks, the effort put forth into exercise will be well worthwhile.

Lastly, remember the importance of having fun. If you try out an exercise and find that you hate it, move on to something else. Or get a partner. Do it any way you can, but make exercise a regular part of your life. You won't be sorry.

Chapter 8:
What Somatoneural Dysfunction is Not

It is Not From a Fungal Infection

One alternative school of thought for fibromyalgia and other types of chronic fatigue is based on ancient Chinese medical theory. Early Chinese practitioners knew of some remedies that helped patients, but had no idea how they worked. They were faced with the task of treating patients and coming up with a rational explanation for the treatments and spoke of the yin and yang. They said that people became ill because evil humors and toxins invaded the body and created disharmony among the forces that kept one healthy.

It must be re-emphasized that 30-35% of all patients with Somatoneural Dysfunction will get better within three months without any specific treatment. Health care practitioners (from medical doctors to aromatherapists) like to take credit for these "cures" and have discovered dozens of explanations as to why the patient gets better. Simple education, diet, and exercise programs will help up to 50% of SND patients recover without any effort on the part of the medical practitioner other than common sense. The mechanism of recovery is, however, fully from the physical and psychological efforts of the patient.

Practitioners will commonly test for things like fungal organisms in the stool and try to eradicate the fungus with powerful anti-fungal medications and dietary therapy. A review of the literature and human clinical evidence was done in 1996 in Germany and offered the following conclusions:

> "Yeast in stool specimen are due to transient
> or commensal growth in the GI tract. Only
> in immune deficient subjects Candida albicans
> may grow invasively in squamous epithelium...
> systemic therapy does not add benefit to local
> measures. Candida-induced diarrhea in hospital-
> ized patients stops after a few days of nystatin
> treatment. Candida hypersensitivity syndrome
> does not exist, antifungal diet does not eradicate
> yeast. Stool examination for candida is of no
> sense because a positive finding is seen in up to
> 80% of healthy persons (Rosch, 1996)."

The use of a yeast-free and/or sugar-free diet is not associated with significant morbidity, other than the fact that it doesn't taste very good, so I don't argue too much against those who recommend this approach. There has even been debate as to whether fungus in the stool can cause any symptoms at all, as the vast majority of patients are asymptomatic. There may be certain populations of patients that are particularly sensitive to the Candida in their GI tracts and develop diarrheal illness (Levine, 1995), but no evidence has been found to indicate any association between the yeast and Somatoneural Dysfunction.

Antifungal drugs should not be used in SND due to this lack of effectiveness as well as potential toxicity. Short term treatment (one week to three months) with an agent like terbinafine or itraconazole is relatively well tolerated, with an adverse event rate of around 20%. Most of these have been mild and reversible, although a few cases of death due to allergic reactions or liver failure have been reported. Longer-term treatment, which is generally necessary to completely eradicate fungi from a place where they typically take up residence, is much more likely to cause severe side effects and should certainly be avoided.

Leaky Gut Syndrome

Jake Paul Fratkin, OMD (Doctor of Oriental Medicine) describes a syndrome of intestinal inflammation and irritation that allows intestinal "toxins" to leak into the bloodstream. This syndrome, he claims, is the cause of chronic fatigue syndrome, fibromyalgia, irritable bowel syndrome, migraine headaches, rheumatoid arthritis, asthma, food allergy, chronic sinusitis, eczema, and fungal disorders. It is also thought to contribute to the development of PMS (pre-menstrual syndrome), uterine fibroids, and breast lumps. By his estimate, 50% of all chronic human disease can be linked to leaky gut syndrome! (Fratkin, 1999).

He writes that modern use of non-steroidal anti-inflammatory medicines (NSAIDS) and antibiotics have led to this condition. In fact, this part of his theories is true: NSAIDS can lead to intestinal inflammation and ultimately cause ulcers in the protective mucosal lining of the bowels, and antibiotics do eliminate beneficial bacteria that live in the bowel and may cause overgrowth of other harmful bacteria or fungus (such as Candida) or even lead to vitamin deficiencies.

The remainder of his theories run from the absolutely true (the liver plays a major role in detoxifying harmful chemicals that pass through the bloodstream) to the absolutely false the adrenal gland is the "most important organ" in the production of immune system components. Unfortunately, he does not know what these destructive toxins are, and instead hides behind thousand-year old Chinese theory of yin and yang.

We don't know what "IT" is, but "IT" must be causing some imbalance in the forces of yin and yang. Modern physicians, even ones who are Chinese, believe in fact not fantasy to diagnose and treat their patients. In my review of the last 30 years of Chinese medical literature, I can find no reference to "leaky gut syndrome". Fratkin recommends a panel of expensive (and probably worthless) tests to assess for leaky gut syndrome. The mainstays of his diagnostic algorithm are serum tests for food allergy and stool assays to quantify the level of Candida. He sends blood

Table 31 Recommended Tests for Leaky Guy Syndrome
Serum IgG/IgE test for food allergies
Stool Candida levels
Chymotrypsin level
Intestinal permeability test
Anti-chymotrypsin level in stools
Secretory IgA level

samples to a specific laboratory that has experience in checking IgG and IgE levels of anti-bodies in blood samples for specific food patterns.

There is a reason why this is the only laboratory in the country that checks for IgG and IgE levels in the blood: it isn't at all useful. IgE is the antibody involved in the immune response, acting to trigger the cells of the immune response. Levels of IgG are independent of allergy and are only an indication of exposure. They serve no memory purpose to tell whether or not the immune system should be triggered in response to something or not. Patch or skin prick testing is just as accurate at detecting allergy as blood testing and is a lot less expensive. The gold standard to detect food allergy is food challenge testing, which should be performed by an experienced allergist.

Supporters of the leaky gut theory rationalize that these latter tests are not sensitive enough to pick up low-grade levels of allergy that cause intestinal inflammation. If the level of antibody response is not enough to be truly "allergic" and trigger the immune system to respond, why would it cause leakiness in the intestine?

There has never been an association with intestinal inflammation and "leaky gut syndrome". It would stand to reason that patients who actually do have intestinal inflammation (those with ulcers or gastritis) would be more prone to the consequences of gut leakiness, but alas, they're not.

As for Candida, I've already addressed that issue a few pages ago. The presence of Candida in the stool is found in 80% of all people, and the levels have never been shown to correlate with any kind of clinical syndrome unless it gets into the blood, urinary tract, or vaginal area.

The intestinal permeability test is an interesting one. Great Smokies Laboratory has the patient ingest two types of sugars and measures the levels in the urine. Intestinal absorption of sugars is usually either directly proportional to that ingested, as measured by blood levels. Urinary levels are independent of what is absorbed, however. The urinary excretion of sugar is related to how the sugar is used in the body. For example, a diabetic can't use sugar properly, so excess levels tend to be excreted in the urine if the blood levels go above about 240 mg/dL. Other sugars are dealt with in the same way, what is needed is kept, what is not is excreted. Nothing to do with the intestinal lining since it is completely permeable to sugar via receptor transport.

Sugar absorption is abnormal in some specific medical conditions. After small bowel resection, for example, permeability is changed dramatically to compensate for lost absorbable surface area (D'Antiga, 1999). Sugar levels in the urine can be altered in malabsorption, such as in a disease called celiac sprue. This illness results from damage to the intestine by ingestion of gluten-containing products in the diet. This is very similar in theory to the leaky gut syndrome, except in this case the inflammation caused by allergy to gluten makes the intestine less permeable not more permeable, the direct opposite of what leaky gut supporters claim.

The other tests are even less likely to be of any diagnostic purpose. Chymotrypsin is produced by the pancreas, but is not a good marker for pancreatic insufficiency because it is an acute-phase reactant. Levels rise during any kind of illness, inflammation, or stress. Lipase and amylase are much more specific markers of pancreatic malfunction (Aggarwal, 1990) and are not abnormal in Somatoneural Dysfunction (nor apparently, in leaky gut syndrome). Fratkin then claims that chymotrypsin abnormalities are indicative of imbalance in splenic qi. Why the spleen is involved in this theory is theoretically a bit murky since chymotrypsin has nothing to do with splenic function and would simply pass through on occasion like every acute phase reactant (Wang, 1998).

I cannot even begin to imagine why the levels of anti-chymotrypsin antibodies in the stool would be of any relevance. Fratkin claims they are directly proportional to the level of inflammation in the intestine, but they are not consistently increased in true diseases of gut inflammation (inflammatory bowel disease or peptic ulcer disease to name a few). Furthermore, they would be increased in other inflammatory conditions (lupus, rheumatoid arthritis, and many others) so could potentially lead to serious misdiagnosis and mistreatment.

Lastly, secretory IgA is purported to be very low in the stool of patients with leaky gut syndrome, thus indicating reduced immune function. Secretory IgA is simply a measure of immune reactivity at mucosal sites (intestines, bronchial airways, mouth, etc). This can be due to microbes or allergy particles. Why then would a patient with overgrowth of fungus (Candida) in the gut have low levels of IgA? It should be high. And if there is so much inflammation going on, shouldn't that stimulate the immune system too? Not, apparently, in the world of the leaky gut proponents who often seem to make up their own laws of biology to fit their erroneous theories.

The recommended treatment approaches to leaky gut syndrome are also fraught with inaccuracies and potentially harmful remedies. The anti-Candida and food allergy diet is probably not harmful, but is extremely hard to adhere to. It requires elimination of dairy products, eggs, gluten-containing grains (wheat, rye, oats), corn, beans, soy, and nuts, in addition to any other foods one is "allergic" to.

After food allergies are dealt with, Candida is eradicated from the stool with a four-month treatment program of oral nystatin (one million units, three times a day). Unfortunately, permanent eradication of Candida is probably not possible. In immunosuppressed patients, nystatin has been used to decrease the risk of systemic Candida infection (during intensive chemotherapy for example), but the fungus simply comes back after treatment is stopped (Blaschke-Hellmessen, 1996). Fortunately, nystatin therapy is relatively safe, with gastrointestinal upset the only likely side effect.

I also find it odd that these authors say that antibiotic use kills of normal gut bacteria, which leads to leaky gut from inflammation, yet they recommend killing off normal fungus with antifungal agents. Fratkin's use of traditional Chinese medicines and herbal remedies to restore normal function of the liver, kidney, and spleen may have some merit. At this time, however, no benefit has ever been shown by research data and thus cannot be recommended. The expense of such therapy is extremely high and neither safety, nor efficacy has been established.

I've found that the leaky gut theory has capitalized on the fact that many patients with these syndromes recover on their own and have made do with a semi-plausible explanation. That the explanation is related to an "infection" simply is the simplest approach for patients to understand. Dr. Fratkin's success with patients probably has much more to do with a placebo effect and a kind and caring approach to treatment than anything else. At some point, a randomized, controlled trial of antifungal agents in SND might be considered, but at this point there isn't even enough evidence to suggest success to bother trying a study.

Chiari I Malformation

Much attention has been made recently about the link between fibromyalgia/chronic fatigue and surgery to correct a Chiari I Malformation and or Cervical Spinal Stenosis. A Chiari I Malformation is a congenital condition that affects the base of the skull where it joins the spinal column. This abnormality causes a protrusion of the cerebellum through the base of the skull and into the spinal canal. It was originally described by a German pathologist named, not surprisingly, Chiari in 1890.

Symptoms of Chiari I Malformation may include: headache, neck pain, dizziness, vision problems, balance problems, muscle weakness, difficulty swallowing, gagging, choking, and sleep apnea. Obviously, there is a significant overlap with fibromyalgia and other types of Somatoneural Dysfunction. However, trigger and tender points and widespread pain are not usually characteristic of Chiari malformation and Chiari patients almost always have identifiable neurologic deficits on clinical examination (Milhorat, 1999).

The bottom line is that a small portion of fibromyalgia patients may really have Chiari I malformation instead. This doesn't mean that Chiari I malformation has anything to do with SND, but is really just another disorder to keep in mind when ruling out other processes before establishing the diagnosis of SND. Patients with characteristic headache and neck pain patterns, especially with neurologic findings, merit MRI scanning of the brain and cervical spine to assess for a potentially correctable neurosurgical problem.

Others?

There are probably dozens of other potential "causes" and "cures" for types of Somatoneural Dysfunction. These range from guaifenesin (to correct abnormalities in phosphate metabolism) to transfer factor 6 (to enhance immune function) to a myriad of simple herbal combinations marketed with trade names to entice SND sufferers (CFS Relief or Fibro-Be-Gone or whatever). I'll leave the discussion of these and many other treatments, both effective and ineffective, in my next book. For now, suffice it to say that you should always seek professional guidance when buying any product that promises benefit without evidence. Check with your doctor!

Epilogue

Figure 1: Dermatome map

Figure 2: Tender point chart, enclosed in "Figure 2.pdf", copyright J. Christian Hoffman. Printed with permission

Figure 3: Sleep EEG recording

Afterword

Many of the works I have seen relating to fibromyalgia, chronic fatigue syndrome, and the other related disorders described in the preceding pages discuss treatment options as they go along.

"Take drug X for muscle spasm"

"Take herb B for insomnia"

"Use a TENS unit for numbness"

"Take these vitamins, well, just for the heck of it"

And so on. Soon, you're head starts to spin, your medicine cabinet looks like the back shelf at the local pharmacy, and your wallet feels much lighter than usual. Dr. Starlanyl's fine book lists over thirty drug treatments that have been advocated in fibromyalgia, most without any suggestion or recommendation for their effectiveness or use. Dr. Teitlebaum's book lists 131 treatments! Dozens of other treatment options exist and the possible combinations for a given patient can be mind-boggling.

Rather than throw all of this at you, my reader, at once, I have opted to take the treatment section of this book and publish it separately. If you have read this book and you have determined that what I have said sounds true and the patients I have described sound like you or someone you know, then you can move on to the second book. If you are still skeptical, by all means continue to educate yourself and look around for what other theories are out there. Come back if you choose, or good luck if you don't (but please be careful out there because it can be dangerous on your own".

Part 2 divides treatments into symptom types and simply lists and describes each possible treatment in the relative order of effectiveness. Some treatments have a lot of clinical research and data to support their use, I may have personally found others useful in my practice, and others may be useful only in theory and should be reserved if the better studied options have failed. I will also tell you why I think these treatments work. You have to believe in the treatment to get the most benefit.

Unlike just about all other works on this topic, I will also spend a lot of time telling you what treatments don't work as well. I'll back up my opinions in scientific studies and tell you why I am biased if the need arises. I will also tell you whether they just don't work (and will just hurt you in the wallet) or whether they are dangerous (and will hurt you in other ways).

I hope you'll consider picking up Part 2 soon, since I feel we've only just begun.

Conclusions

I am hopeful that you now have a better understanding of Somatoneural Dysfunction, including fibromyalgia, chronic fatigue syndrome, and a host of other similar ailments. Several "take home" messages should by now become apparent.

1) SND is not a psychiatric disturbance, although psychological factors play an important role in the course of the illness
2) You are not alone. Millions of people of all shapes and sizes around the world suffer from SND
3) The involvement of a physician and multidisciplinary medical team is critical to receiving proper treatment
4) SND is manageable and should not result in disability if treated properly
5) There is strength within each patient that can help overcome the detrimental effects of the syndrome

We have also learned that the medical community is just now beginning to develop an understanding of SND and that the efforts of researchers like I. Jon Russell in San Antonio, Robert Bennett in Portland, Daniel Clauw at Georgetown, and many others will have a tremendous impact on battling the spectrum of illness seen in SND in the next decade.

We must realize, however, that many in the medical community are not supportive of such research and treatment efforts and that, unfortunately, the fringes of medicine and alternative medicine are all too willing to take your hard earned money in exchange for unproven and unrealistic treatments. I highly recommend that every "new advance" be viewed with a great deal of skepticism until proven as fact by a preponderance of sound medical evidence.

We have barely scratched the surface of therapy for SND. Full treatment involves a basis of diet and exercise to recondition the body, management of detrimental psychological events in order to recondition the mind, and the alleviation of symptoms in order to improve quality of life and to better allow such reconditioning. In part two, we will examine such treatment options in great detail, including assessment of what works, what might work, and what doesn't work. And, as always, we will answer the question "why" and "why not".

About the Author

Dr. Martin A. Duclos is a practicing internal medicine physician in Pittsburgh, Pennsylvania. He works for Highmark Blue Cross and Blue Shield in the practice of Edward Jew III and Associates with four partners. In addition to this thriving clinical practice, Dr. Duclos is appointed as a Clinical Instructor in Medicine at the University of Pittsburgh School of Medicine and holds staff appointments at several area hospitals. He is a former delegate to the Pennsylvania Medical Society and writes for the Allegheny County Medical Society about issues facing physicians today. A graduate of New York Medical College, Dr. Duclos started his medical career at St. George's University School of Medicine in Grenada and finished a residency in Primary Care Internal Medicine at the University of Pittsburgh Medical Center. He also holds a bachelor's degree in Neuroscience from the University of Rochester, where he also worked as a laboratory assistant for projects designed by MacArthur Foundation Scholar, Dr. David Felten

Appendix

How To Find Me on the Internet

<u>Interactive MD</u>

I have found that the internet is an excellent portal for exchanging information across the country and over the world. However, I have also found that it is a portal for anyone to say anything they want, right or wrong. In the field of health care this can be a dangerous practice. Often, desperate patients encounter unscrupulous entrepreneurs who prey on them, offering hope, but taking their money without giving anything useful in return.

So I developed a web site (like everyone else in the world, it seems) and sponsored a newsgroup to answer questions from patients before they go off and waste time and money on bogus, or at least unproven, remedies. It also has allowed me to disseminate information to larger groups of patients. Unfortunately, there isn't enough space on the World Wide Web to say all that needs to be said, so this book was written in addition.

I would encourage every reader to come and join our club if they have internet access. It's real easy. Go to <u>http://www.yahoo.com</u> and sign up for a free membership. Under the heading of "groups", y'all can find me at "Fibromyalgia Medical Group". I will be available to answer questions about the information in this book and any other questions you might have. Depending on the demand, I am usually to answer questions personally within a week's time.

Of course, the information contained in this book and on my web pages does not replace the typical doctor-patient relationship, but merely supplements it. I would also gladly consult with your physicians to educate and inform them and to further the medical communities understanding of these disorders. I would like you the reader to feel as if, along with the paper and ink contained in this book, you are getting a personal health advisor for your hard-earned dollars. If you do not have internet access, no problem, I still remember how to read mail the old fashioned way.

References

Abbey SE, Garfinkel PE. Neurasthenia and the chronic fatigue syndrome: the role of culture in the making of a diagnosis. Am Journal of Psychiatry 1991; 148:1638-1646.

Ahles TA, Khan SA, Yunus MB, et al. Psychiatric status of primary fibromyalgia and rheumatoid arthritis patients and nonpain controls: A blinded comparison of DSM-III diagnoses. American Journal of Psychiatry, 1991; 148:1721-1726.

Agarwal N, Pitchumoni CS, Sivaprasad AV. Evaluating tests for pancreatitis. American Journal of Gastroenterology, 1990; 85(4):356-366.

Albrecht RM, Oliver VL, Poskanzer DC. Epidemic neuromyasthenia: an outbreak in a convent in New York State. JAMA 1964; 187:904-907.

Ang D, Wilke WS. Diagnosis, etiology, and therapy of fibromyalgia. Comprehensive Therapy 1999; 25(4):221-228.

Angrilli A, Mini A, Mucha RF, et al. The influence of low blood pressure and baroreceptor activity on pain responses. Physiology and Behavior, 1997; 62:391.

Barr IR, et al. Testing the neural sensitization and kindling hypothesis for illness from low levels of environmental chemicals. Environmental Health Perspectives, 1997; 105(suppl 2):539-547.

Barsky AJ, Borus JF. Functional somatic syndromes. Annals of Internal Medicine, 1999; 130(11):910-921.

Bates DW, Schmitt W, Buchwald D, Ware NC, Lee J, Thoyer E, et. al. Prevalence of fatigue and chronic fatigue syndrome in a primary care practice. Archives of Internal Medicine 1993; 153:2759-65.

Beard G. Cited by: Rosenberg CE. The place of George M. Beard in nineteenth-century psychiatry. Bull Hist Med 1962; 36:245-259.

Bell D. Chronic fatigue syndrome update. Postgraduate Medicine 1994; 96(4):73-82.

Bell KM, Cookfair D, Bell DS. Risk factors associated with chronic fatigue syndrome in a cluster of pediatric cases. Review of Infectious Diseases, 1991; 13(suppl 1):S32-38.

Bennett RM. Emerging concepts in the neurobiology of chronic pain: evidence of abnormal sensory processing in fibromyalgia. Mayo Clinic Proceedings, 1999; 74(4):385-98.

Blaschke-Hellmessen R, Buchman H,Schwarze R. Effect of orally administered polyene antimycotics on the intestinal colonization with yeasts: possibilities and limitations. Mycoses, 1996; 39(suppl 1):33-39.

Boyce PM, Koloski NA, Talley NJ. Irritable bowel syndrome according to varying criteria: are the new Rome II criteria unnecessarily restrictive for research and practice? American Journal of Gastroenterology. 2000; 95(11):3176-3183.

Briggs NC, Levine PH. A comparative review of systemic and neurological symptomatology in 12 outbreaks collectively described as chronic fatigue syndrome, epidemic neuromyasthenia, or myalgic encephalomyelitis. Clinical Infectious Disease 1994; 18(suppl 1):S32-42.

Buchwald, D. Fibromyalgia and chronic fatigue syndrome. Rheumatic Disease Clinics of North America 1996; 22(2):219-239.

Buskila D, Neumann L. Fibromyalgia syndrome (FM) and nonarticular tenderness in relatives of patients with FM. Journal of Rheumatology, 1997; 24:941.

Cheuvront SN. The zone diet and athletic performance. Sports Medicine, 1999; 27(4):213-228.

Clauw DJ, Sabol M, Radulovic D, Wilson B, Katz P, Baraniuk J. Serum neuropeptides in patients with both fibromyalgia and chronic fatigue syndrome. Journal of Musculoskeletal Pain, 1995; 3(Suppl 1): 79.

Cope H, David A, Pelosi A, Mann A. Predictors of chronic "postviral" fatigue. Lancet, 1994; 344:864-868.

Cote KA, Moldofsky H. Sleep and cognitive performance in fibromylagia. The Journal of Rheumatology, 1997; 24(10):2014-2023.

Cullen MR, Redlich CA. Significance of individual sensitivity to chemicals: elucidation of host susceptibility by use of biomarkers in environmental health research. Clinical Chemistry. 1995; 41(12 pt 2):1809-1813.

D'Antiga L, Dhawan A, Davenport M, et al. Intestinal absorption and permeability on pediatric short-bowel syndrome: a pilot study. Journal of Pediatric Gastroenterology and Nutrition, 1999; 29(5):588-593.

Demitrack MA, Crawford LJ. Evidence for and pathophysiologic implications of hypothalamic-pituitary-adrenal axis dysregulation in fibromyalgia and chronic fatigue syndrome. Annals of the New York Academy of the Sciences 1994; 685-694.

Dietert RR, Hedge AA. Chemical sensitivity and the immune system: a paradigm to approach potential immune involvement. Neurotoxicology, 1998; 19(2):253-257.

Drossman DA, Sandler RS, McKee DC, et al. Bowel patterns among subjects not seeking health care: use of a questionnaire to identify a population with bowel dysfunction. Gastroenterology, 1982; 83:529.

Durstine JL, Painter P, Franklin BA, et al. Physical activity for the chronically ill and disabled. Sports Medicine. 2000; 30(3):207-219.

Escalante A, Fischbach M. Musculoskeletal manifestations, pain, and quality of life in Persian Gulf War veterans referred for rheumatologic evaluation. Journal of Rheumatology, 1998; 25(11):2228-2235.

Everson MP, Kotler S, Blackburn WD Jr. Stress and immune dysfunction in Gulf War veterans. Annals of the New York Academy of Science, 1999; 876:413-418.

Fiatarone MA, O'Neill EF, Ryan ND, et al. Exercise training and nutritional supplementation for physical frailty in very elderly people. New England Journal of Medicine, 1994; 30:1769-1775.

Fukuda K, et. al. The chronic fatigue syndrome: a comprehensive approach to its definition and study. Annals of Internal Medicine 1994; 121:953-959.

Garfinkel MS, Schumacher HR Jr, Husain A, Levy M, Reshetar RA. Evaluation of yoga based regimen for treatment of osteosrthritis of the hands. Journal of Rheumatology, 1994; 21(12): 341-2343.

Garfinkel MS, Singhal A, Katz WA, Allan DA, Rashetar R, Schumacher HR Jr. Yoga-based intervention for carpal tunnel syndrome: a randomized trial. JAMA, 1998, 280(18):1601-1603.

Glaser R, Kiecolt-Glaser JK. Stress-associated immune modulation: relevance to viral infections and chronic fatigue syndrome. The American Journal of Medicine 1998; 105 (3A):35S-42S.

Goldenberg D. An overview of psychological studies in fibromyalgia. Journal of Rheumatology, 1989; 16(suppl 19):12-13.

Gots RE. Multiple chemical sensitivities: public policy. Journal of Clinical Toxicology. 1995; 33(2):111-113.

Hawley DJ, Wolfe F. Depression is not more common in rheumatoid arthritis: a ten-year longitudinal study of 6153 patients with rheumatic disease. Journal of Rheumatology, 1993; 20:2025-2031.

Haynes RB, Sackett DL, Taylor DW, Gibson ES, Johnson AL. Increased absenteeism from work after detection and labeling of hypertensive patients. New England Journal of Medicine, 1978; 299:741-744.

Henderson DA. Reflections on epidemic neuromyastheni (chronic fatigue syndrome). Clinical Infectious Diseases 1994; 18(suppl):S3-S6.

Hoare M. The Resolution journal of Johann Reinhold Forster: London: Hakluyt Society, 1982.

Holmes GP, Kaplan JE, Gantz NM, Komaroff AL, Schonberger LB, Straus SE, et al. Chronic fatigue syndrome: a working case definition. Annals of Internal Medicine 1988; 108:387-389.

Inbal R, et.al. Collateral sprouting in skin and sensory recovery after nerve injury in man. Pain. 1987; 28:141.

Ismail K, Everitt B, Blatchley N. Is there a Gulf War syndrome? Lancet, 1999; 352(9148):179-182.

Jin P. Changes in heart rate, noradrenaline, cortisol, and mood during Tai Chi. Journal of Psychosomatic Research, 1989; 33(2):197-206.

Katon W, Sullivan MD. Depression and chronic medical illness. Journal of Clinical Psychiatry, 1990; 51(suppl):3-11.

Kehrl HR. Laboratory testing of the patient with multiple chemical sensitivity. Environmental Health Perspectives, 1997; 105(suppl 2):443-444.

Kellow JE, Phillips SF. Altered small bowel motility in irritable bowel syndrome is correlated with symptoms. Gastroenterology, 1987; 92:1885.

Kim E. A brief history of chronic fatigue syndrome. JAMA 1994; 272:1070-72.

Klaustmeyer WB, Kraske GK, Lee KG, et al. Allergic and immunologic profile of symptomatic Persian Gulf War veterans. Annals of Allergy, Asthma, and Immunology, 1998; 80(3):269-273.

Kroenke K, Wood DR, Mangelsdorff AD, Meier NJ, Powell JB. Chronic fatigue in primary care. Prevalence, patient characteristics, and outcome. JAMA 1988; 206:929-34.

Krueger BR. Restless legs syndrome and periodic movements of sleep. Mayo Clinics Preceedings, 1990; 65:999.

Larson AA, Giovengo SL, et al. Changes in the concentrations of amino acids in the cerebrospinal fluid that correlate with pain in fibromyalgia: implications for nitric oxide pathways. Pain. 2000, 87(2):201-211.

Lasser RB, Bond JH, Levitt MD. The role of abdominal gas in functional abdominal pain. New England Journal of Medicine, 1975; 293:524.

Lax MB, Henneberger PK. Patients with multiple chemical sensitivities in an occupational health clinic: presentation and follow-up. Archives of Environmental Health, 1995; 50:425-31.

Levine J, et al. Candida-associated diarrhea: a syndrome in search of credibility. Clinical Infectious Diseases, 1995; 21(4):881-886.

Levine P. A review of Human Herpesvirus-6 infection. Infections in Medicine 1995; 12(8):395-400.

Levine PH, Snow PG, Ranum BG, et. al. Epidemic neuromyasthenia and chronic fatigue syndrome in West Otago, New Zealand. Achives of Internal Medicine 1997; 157:750-754.

Lewis T. A lecture on vasovagal syncope and the carotid sinus mechanism. British Medical Journal 1932; 1:873-876.

Low PA, Opfer-Gehrking TL, McFee BR, et al. Prospective evaluation of clinical characteristics of orthostatic hypotension. Mayo Clinics Proceedings 1995; 70:617-622.

Lynn RB, Friedman LS. Irritable bowel syndrome: managing the patient with abdominal pain and altered bowel habits. Medical Clinics of North America, 1995; 79(2):373-390.

McCain GA. Fibromyalgia and myofascial pain syndromes. In: Wall PD, Melzack, eds. Textbook of Pain. 3rd edition. Edinburgh: Churchill-Livingstone; 1994:475-493.

McEvedy CP, Beard AW. Royal Free epidemic of 1955: a reconsideration. British Medical Journal 1970; 1:7-11.

McEvedy CP, Beard AW. Concept of benign myalgic encephalomyelitis. British Medical Journal 1970; 1:11-15.

Maixner W, Fillingim RB, Kincaid S, et al. Relationship between pain sensitivity and resting arterial blood pressure in patients with painful temporomandibular disorders. Psychosomatic Medicine, 1997; 59:503.

Martin L, Nutting A, et al. An exercise program in the treatment of fibromyalgia. Journal of Rheumatology. 1996; 23(6):1050-1053.

Maughan RJ, Greenhaff PL, Leiper JB, et al. Diet composition and the performance of high intensity exercise. Journal of Sports Science, 1997; 15(3):265-275.

Mayer EA, Raybould HE. Role of visceral afferent mechanisms in functional bowel disorders. Gastroenterology, 1990; 99:1688.

Meiworm L, Jacob E, et al. Patients with fibromyalgia benefit from aerobic exercise. Clinical Rheumatology. 2000; 19(4):253-257.

Mikalian AJ. Vasomotor rhinitis. Ear, Nose, and Throat. 1989; 68:207.

Mikkelsson M, Latikka P, Kautainen H, Isomeri R, Isomaki H. Muscle and bone pressure pain threshold and pain tolerance in patients fibromyalgia patients and controls. Archives of Disease and Physical Medicine Rehabilitation, 1992; 73:814-818.

Milhorat TH, Chou MW, Trinidad EM, et al. Chiari I malformation redefined: clinical and radiographic findings for 364 symptomatic patients. Journal of Neurosurgery. 1999; 44:1005-1017.

Moldofsky H, Sacrisbrick P, England R, Smyth H. Musculoskeletal symptoms and non-REM sleep disturbance in patients with "fibrositis syndrome" and healthy subjects. Psychosomatic Medicine, 1975; 37: 341-351.

Moldofsky H, Scarisbrick P. Induction of neurasthenic musculoskeletal pain syndrome by selective sleep stage deprivation. Psychosomatic Medicine, 1976; 38:35-44.

Myers MG, Cairns JA, Singer J. The consent form as a possible cause of side effects. Clinical Pharmacological Therapeutics, 1987; 42:250-253.

Paz A, Berry EM. Effect of meal composition on alertness and performance of hospital night-shift workers. Do mood and performance have different determinants. Annals of Nutrition and Metabolism, 1997; 41 (5):291-298.

Perez-Stable EJ, Miranda J, et al. Depression in medical outpatients. Archives of Internal Medicine. 1990; 150:1083-1088.

Pinkowish MD. The best diet for healthy adults. Patient Care, 1999; 33(18):122-142.

Plaisted CS, Lin PH, Ard JD, McCLure ML, Svetkey LP. The effects of dietary patterns on quality of life: a substudy of the Dietary Approaches to Stop Hypertension trial. Journal of the American Dietetic Association, 1999; 99(8 suppl):S84-89.

Pollet C, Natelson BH, Lange G, et al. Medical evaluation of Persian Gulf veterans with fatigue and/or chemical sensitivity. Journal of Medicine, 1998; 29(3):101-113.

Pollock ML, Vincent KR. Resistance training for health. The President's Council on Physical Fitness and Sports Research Digest, 1996, Series 2, Number 8.

Powell P, Bentall RP, et al. Randomised controlled trial of patient education to encourage graded exercise in chronic fatigue syndrome. British Journal of Medicine. 2001; 322(7283):387.

Price RK, North CS, Wessely S, Fraser VJ. Estimating the prevalence of chronic fatigue syndrome and associated symptoms in the community. Public Health Rep 1992; 107:512-22.

Proctor SP, Heeren T, White RF, et al. Health status of Persian Gulf War veterans: self-reported symptoms, environmental exposures and the effect of stress. International Journal of epidemiology, 1998; 27(6):1000-1010.

Ramsey SM. Holistic manual therapy techniques. Primary Care, 1997; 24(4):759-786.

Rechstaffen A. Current perspectives on the function of sleep. Perspectives in Biology and Medicine; 41(3):359-390.

Rosch W. Fungi in feces, fungi in the intestines: therapeutic consequences? Versicherungsmedizin, 1996; 48(6):215-217.

Rosomoff HL, Rosomoff RS. Low back pain: evaluation and management in the primary care setting. The Medical Clinics of North America 1999; 83(3):643-662.

Rowe PC, Calkins H. Neurally mediated hypotension and chronic fatigue syndrome. Annals of Internal Medicine 1998; 105(3A):15S-21S.
St. George, IM. Did Cook's sailors have Tapanui 'flu—chronic fatigue syndrome on the Resolution. New England Journal of Medicine, 1996; 109(1016):15-7

Saper, JR. Headache disorders. The Medical Clinics of North America 1999; 83(3):663-690.

Schweiger A, Parducci A. Nocebo: the psychologic induction of pain. Pavlov Journal of Biological Sciences, 1981; 16:140-143.

Sheffield D, Krittayaphong R, Go BM, et al. The relationship between resting systolic blood pressure and cutaneous pain perception in cardiac patients with angina pectoris and controls. Pain, 1997; 71:249.

Shelokov A, Habel K, Veder E, Walsh W. Epidemic neuromyasthenia: an outbreak of poliomyelitis-like illness in student nurses. New England Journal of Medicine 1957; 257:345-355.

Sigurdsson B, Sigurjonsson J, Sigurdsson JH, Thorkelsson J, Gundmundsson KR. A disease in Iceland simulating poliomyelitis. American Journal of Hygiene 1950; 52:222-228.

Smythe H.Fibrositis syndrome: a historical perspective.Journal of Rheumatology 1989(suppl 19); 16:2-6.

Snape WJ, Carlson GM, Cohen S. Colonic myoelectric activation the irritable bowel syndrome. Gastroenterology, 1976; 20:326.

Sorensen J, et al. Fibromyalgia-are there different mechanisms in the processing of pain? A double-blind, crossover comparison of analgesic drugs. Journal of rheumatology, 1997; 24(8):1615-1621.

Spiegel D. Effect of psychosocial treatment on survival of patients with metastatic breast cancer. Lancet, 1989; II:888-891.

Spitzer RL, Williams JBW, Kroenke K, et al. Utility of a new procedure for diagnosing mental disorders in primary care. JAMA 1994; 272(22):1749-1757.

Thomas KQ. The mind-body connection: granny was right after all. The Rochester Review 1997; 59:N3.

Touchette N. Research brief: estrogen signals a novel route to pain relief. Journal of the National Institute of Health Research. 1993; 5:53.

Trotto N. Exercise for optimum health. Patient Care, 1999; 33(18):97-112.

Vassallo M, Camilleri M, Phillips SF, et al. Transit through the proximal colon influences stool weight in the irritable bowel syndrome. Gastroenterology, 1992; 102:102.

Wallace DJ. Fibromyalgia: unusual historical aspects and new pathogenic insights. The Mount Sinai Journal of Medicine 1984; 51:124-130.

Wang XC, Strauss KI, Ha QN, et al. Chymotrypsin gene expression in rat peripheral organs. Cell and Tissue Research, 1998; 292(2):345-354.

Wells AS, Read NW, Laugharne JD, Ahluwalia NS. Alterations in mood after changing to a low-fat diet. British Journal of Nutrition, 1998; 79(1):23-30.

Whitehead WE, Bosmajian L, Zonderman AB, et al. Symptoms of psychological distress associated with irritable bowel syndrome: comparisons of community and medical clinic samples. Gastroenterology, 1988; 95:709.

Winfield JB. Pain in fibromyalgia. Rheumatic Disease Clinics of North America, 1999: 25(1):55-79.

Wolfe F, et.al. Service utilization and costs in fibromyalgia. Arthritis and Rheumatism 1997; 40:1565-70.

Wolfe F, Ross K, Anderson J, Russel IJ, Hebert L. The prevalence and characteristics of fibromyalgia in the general population. Arthritis and Rheumatism 1995; 38:19-28.

Wolfe F, Simmons DG, Fricton J, et al. The fibromyalgia and myofascial pain syndromes: a preliminary study of tender points and trigger points in persons with fibromyalgia, myofascial pain syndrome, and no disease. Journal of Rheumatology. 1992: 19:944.

Wood C. Mood change and perceptions of vitality: a comparison of the effects of relaxation, visualization, and yoga. J R Soc Med, 1993; 86 (5):254-258

Woolf CJ, Shortland P, Coggershall RA. Peripheral nerve injury triggers sprouting of myelinated afferents. Nature. 1992; 355:75.

Yunus MB, et al. Plasma tryptophan and other amino acids in primary fibromyalgia: a controlled study. Journal of Rheumatology, 1992; 19:90-94.

Bibliography

Ader Robert, Felten David L, Cohen Nicholas. eds. Psychoneuroimmunology, second edition. New York: Academic, 2001. 3rd edition. San Diego. Academic Press.

Principles of Neural Science. Edited by Eric J. Kandel, James H. Schwartz, Thomas M. Jessell. 4th edition. McGraw-Hill Health Professions Division. New york. 2000

Bierce, Ambrose. The devil's dictionary. New York: Dover Publications, 1993

Guyton, Arthur C. Textbook of medical physiology. 10th Ed. Philadelphia: Saunders, 2000.

Harrison's Principles of Internal Medicine. 2001. Eugene Braunwald, et.al. 15th edition. McGraw-Hill. New York

Kaplan and Sadock's Comprehensive Textbook of Psychiatry. Editors Benjamain J. Sadock and Virginia A. Sadock. 7th Edition. Philadelphia. Lippincott Williams & Wilkins. 2000

Robins' Pathological Basis of Disease. Ramsey S. Cotran, Vinay Kumar. Tucker Collins. Philadelphia. Saunders. 5th edition. 1999.

Popper, Sir Karl Raimund, Eccles John C: The Self and its Brain, Springer-Verlag, 1977. New York.

Starlanyl DJ, Copeland ME. Fibromyalgia & Chronic Myofascial Pain Syndrome. New York. MJF Books. 1998.

Diagnostic and Statistic Manual of Mental Disorders: DSM-IV-TR. 4th edition, text revision. Wshington, DC. American Psychiatric Association.

Sears Barry, Lawren William. Zone: a dietary roadmap. Regan Books, 1995. New York.

Jake Paul Fratkin. Personal correspondence. More information can be found through http://www.gsdl.com

Jacob Teitlebaul. From fatigued to fantastic: a proven program to regain vibrant health, based on a new scientific study showing effective treatment for fibromyalgia and chronic fatigue. 2001. Avery. New York.

What your doctor may not tell you about fibromyalgia: the revolutionary treatment that can reverse the disease. R. Paul St. Armand and Claudia Craig Marek. New York. Warner Books. 1999.

Center for Disease Control. Guidelines for diagnosis of chronic fatigue syndrome. This and a wealth of related information can be found at http://www.cdc.gov/ncidod/diseases.cfs

0-595-24849-7

LaVergne, TN USA
20 December 2010

209522LV00001B/89/A